Postural Correction

Hands-On Guides for Therapists

Jane Johnson, MCSP, MSc

Human Kinetics

Library of Congress Cataloging-in-Publication Data

Johnson, Jane, 1965- , author.
Postural correction / Jane Johnson.
   p. ; cm. -- (Hands-on guides for therapists)
Includes bibliographical references.
I. Title. II. Series: Hands-on guides for therapists.
[DNLM: 1. Posture--physiology. 2. Musculoskeletal Diseases--therapy. 3. Musculoskeletal Manipulations--methods. 4. Spinal Curvatures--therapy. WE 104]
RA781.5
613.7'8--dc23

                  2015018860

ISBN: 978-1-4925-0712-3 (print)

The web addresses cited in this text were current as of July 2015, unless otherwise noted.

Acquisitions Editor: Chris Wright; **Developmental Editor:** Judy Park; **Associate Managing Editor:** Shevone Myrick; **Copyeditor:** Jan Feeney; **Permissions Manager:** Dalene Reeder; **Graphic Designer:** Dawn Sills; **Cover Designer:** Keith Blomberg; **Photograph (cover):** Neil Bernstein, © Human Kinetics; **Photographs (interior):** Neil Bernstein; © Human Kinetics unless otherwise noted. Figures 1.1, 1.2, 1.3, 3.1, 3.4b, 3.7, 3.8, 3.11b, 4.1, 4.5, 4.7b, 5.1a, 5.1c, 5.4c, 6.2a, 7.3c, 7.7c, 7.13a, 7.13c, 8.1, 8.3a, 8.4c, 8.6c, 8.9c, 8.12c, 8.15, 8.17e, 9.4b, 9.10b, 9.10c, 10.1, and 10.2 courtesy of Emma Kelly Photography; **Photo Asset Manager:** Laura Fitch; **Visual Production Assistant:** Joyce Brumfield; **Photo Production Manager:** Jason Allen; **Art Manager:** Kelly Hendren; **Associate Art Manager:** Alan L. Wilborn; **Illustrations:** © Human Kinetics; **Printer:** Versa Press

Special thanks to Douglas Nelson, LMT, for his expertise as the massage therapist in the photographs.

Printed in the United States of America   10 9 8 7 6 5 4 3

The paper in this book is certified under a sustainable forestry program.

Human Kinetics
P.O. Box 5076
Champaign, IL 61825-5076
Website: www.HumanKinetics.com

In the United States, email info@hkusa.com or call 800-747-4457.
In Canada, email info@hkcanada.com.
In the United Kingdom/Europe, email hk@hkeurope.com.

For information about Human Kinetics' coverage in other areas of the world,
please visit our website: **www.HumanKinetics.com**

Contents

PART III   Correcting the Pelvis and Lower Limb

PART IV   Correcting the Shoulder and Upper Limb

Massage may be one of the oldest therapies still used today. At present more therapists than ever before are practicing an ever-expanding range of massage techniques. Many of these techniques are taught through massage schools and within degree courses. Our need now is to provide the best clinical and educational resources that will enable massage therapists to learn the required techniques for delivering massage therapy to clients. Human Kinetics has developed the Hands-On Guides for Therapists series with this in mind.

The Hands-On Guides for Therapists series provides specific tools of assessment and treatment that fall well within the realm of massage therapists but may also be useful for other bodyworkers, such as osteopaths and fitness instructors. Each book in the series is a step-by-step guide to delivering the techniques to clients. Each book features a full-colour interior packed with photos illustrating every technique. Tips provide handy advice to help you adjust your technique.

You might be using a book from the Hands-On Guides for Therapists series to obtain the required skills to help you pass a course or to brush up on skills you learned in the past. You might be a course tutor looking for ways to make massage therapy come alive with your students. This series provides easy-to-follow steps that will make the transition from theory to practice seem effortless. The Hands-On Guides for Therapists series is an essential resource for all those who are serious about massage therapy.

As part of the Hands-On Guides for Therapists, *Postural Correction* is intended for use by professionals who use hands-on skills as part of their treatment. If you are a soft tissue therapist or exercise professional, this book will help you to use your skills of massage and stretching along with simple exercises to help correct posture in your clients, should this be one of your treatment aims. Student physiotherapists, osteopaths, sports therapists and chiropractors will eventually become highly skilled in helping their clients to overcome postural problems. As a student, you too may find the simple descriptions used in *Postural Correction* support your ongoing understanding of the musculoskeletal system. If you are a teacher of yoga or Pilates, you may also benefit from learning how positions or movements you employ in your class might affect the posture of your students. As a result of reading this material, you may gain ideas for structuring programmes to help address specific postural problems.

Whatever your discipline, you are likely to have some of the skills described in *Postural Correction,* but you may not yet know how best to use these skills to bring about postural change. This book informs, reminds and inspires you to help correct posture whether locally at a joint or globally in the entire body.

Postural Correction covers the 30 most common postural formations you are likely to observe in the spine, pelvis, upper limb and lower limb and provides guidance on what you can do as a therapist to help correct each posture. It also presents what your clients with these postures may do for themselves, a crucial component of postural correction. Some postural deviations are the result of habitual ways of resting or using the body, and the information regarding what a client may do for oneself will therefore help your clients to manage and change posture.

The 10 spinal postures covered in this book are increased cervical lordosis, lateral flexion of the head and neck, forward head posture, rotation of the head, kyphosis, flatback (in the thoracic region), rotated thorax, hyperlordosis (increased lumbar lordosis), hypolordosis (decreased lumbar lordosis) and scoliosis. The four most common pelvic postures covered are anterior pelvic tilt, posterior pelvic tilt, pelvic rotation and laterally tilted pelvis.

The 10 common lower-limb postures covered are internal rotation of the hips, genu recurvatum (hyperextension at the knee), genu flexum (flexion at the knee), genu varum (bowlegs), genu valgum (knock knees), tibial torsion, flatfoot (pes planus), high arches in the feet (pes caves), pronation in the foot (pes valgus) and supination in the foot (pes varus).

The six shoulder and upper-limb postures covered are protracted scapula, elevated shoulder, winged scapula, internally rotated humerus, flexed elbows and hyperextended elbows.

Accompanying each of the 30 postures is a description and, in most cases, a photograph giving an example of that particular posture. An overview box lists which muscles are shortened and which are lengthened. For each posture there is a list of ideas. These are presented as bulleted lists under the headings What You Can Do as a Therapist and What Your Client Can Do. Many of the ideas are illustrated with photographs.

As part of the Hands-On Guides for Therapists series, the techniques described here focus on those available to most therapists, particularly massage therapists, and are therefore primarily concerned with the lengthening of shortened tissues in order to help realign body parts. Techniques vary for each posture you may attempt to correct and could include deep tissue massage, simple passive stretch, soft tissue release, deactivation of a trigger point or gentle traction of a limb. Active stretches and resting postures the client may use are illustrated. Tips are provided on the positioning of your client to help facilitate your use of these techniques during treatment, and information on gaining rapport and enhancing engagement with postural correction will help you in your sessions with clients. The techniques described in *Postural Correction* are a valuable adjunct to any joint-manipulative techniques that might be used by qualified physiotherapists, osteopaths and chiropractors.

Postural Correction includes information about those postures that are difficult to correct using the skills employed by massage therapists. Good examples of such postures are scoliosis, genu valgum (knock knees) and genu varum (bow legs), where simply stretching soft tissues and strengthening weak ones are not sufficient for changing underlying bony anatomy. Nevertheless, these postural forms are included along with ideas and suggestions because it is important to know where you are limited as a therapist.

All therapists know that the interconnectedness of human anatomy makes it difficult to separate one part of the musculoskeletal system from another. For example, the neck may affect the lumbar spine; the feet may affect the pelvis; the shoulders affect the wrists and hands. In an ideal world, we would work holistically to bring about complete body alignment, but the realities of life and the limitation of treatment time mean that it is common for us as therapists to address problems in one part of the body at a time. In *Postural Correction,* I hope you will forgive me for presenting material in a compartmentalized manner. With this format you can quickly refer to the section of the book that you believe will be most helpful in your treatment for a particular client.

Material in *Postural Correction* is organized into four parts. The two chapters in part I, Getting Started With Postural Correction, provide the rationale for helping your clients to change their posture and give an overview on the methods suggested in later chapters. Each of the four chapters in part II, Correcting the Spine, focuses on a specific part of the spine and offers explanations on correcting the posture affecting that particular part. Part III, Correcting the Pelvis and Lower Limb, contains two chapters dealing with the pelvis, hip, knee, ankle and foot. Finally, there are two chapters in part IV, Correcting the Shoulder and Upper Limb.

Postural Correction is an ideal volume to accompany *Postural Assessment* and provides insight into how techniques described in *Deep Tissue Massage*, *Therapeutic Stretching* and *Soft Tissue Release* may help you when working with clients wishing to bring about postural change.

PART I

Getting Started With Postural Correction

If you have been using the *Hands-On Guide to Postural Assessment* it is likely that you have started to make notes about the posture of some of your clients and have been wondering what you can do to help change postures that deviate from the norm. Before examining how you might intervene to correct a client's posture, you need to begin with an overview: the why and the how of postural correction. Why should you bother to help a client correct posture? Should you do this for aesthetic reasons or to affect how the client functions and feels? How, in general terms, is posture corrected? Does it require therapeutic intervention? If so, in what way? Starting with these simple questions establishes an understanding of the principles underlying postural correction.

Introduction
to Postural Correction

Learning Outcomes

After reading this chapter, you should be able to do the following:

- Give examples of body structures affected by malalignment.
- State the possible consequences of such malalignment and how these structures could be affected.
- Give examples of the kinds of clients who might be susceptible to malalignment and who might benefit from postural correction.
- Give examples of contraindications to and cautions for postural correction.

This chapter helps you to get started by touching on the causes of postural malalignment and the consequences it might have on bones, muscles, joints and ligaments. Appreciating the way that these structures change when posture is altered will help you understand postural correction and the techniques that are described in chapter 2. Examples of the kinds of clients who might benefit from postural correction are included.

A NOTE ON EFFECTIVENESS OF TECHNIQUE

Whilst this book outlines the rationale for the correction of certain postures, it was not written with the intention of convincing you to change the posture of your clients. Rather, it provides ideas on how postural change might be achieved *once the decision has been made* that changing posture might be beneficial. It is challenging to offer suggestions for the correction of posture when there are no protocols to follow. There are few textbooks on the subject of postural correction; this might be because it is scary for a clinician to put one's professional neck on the line by suggesting a treatment that is not supported by robust evidence. We do not yet know which techniques are most effective at bringing about postural change. We do not know whether massage and stretching of shortened tissues, for example, are as effective or more effective than strengthening muscles or altering habitual postural patterns to help realign body parts. As bodyworkers, we live in a world in which evidence-based practice is not only encouraged, but experimental practice is discouraged. References are included wherever possible, but do not expect the text to be littered with these.

There is scant information on many of the postures covered and little information available on the effectiveness of techniques suggested. Although the techniques offered are not foolproof, they are based on sound experience. My hope in presenting this material to you is twofold: I hope that some readers will experiment with the ideas presented here and that the results will ultimately benefit their clients. My rationale for suggesting this is that you are, after all, not laypersons but informed practitioners; as such you are unlikely to deliver a treatment that is harmful. I also hope that some readers will be inspired to investigate selected techniques, perhaps collaborating on research into their effectiveness. Whether reading this encourages you to write up a case study or inspires you to embark on a larger piece of work, sharing your findings will contribute to our knowledge on this subject. One day we will have far greater information about which postures contribute to pain, which postural correction methods are best used to decrease postural-related pain and whether some of the techniques inherent to postural correction can be used prophylactically to reduce the likelihood of postural-related symptoms developing in the first place.

Causes of Postural Malalignment

Have you ever observed a person using the same mannerisms or standing in the same pose as one of that person's parents or grandparents? Have you noticed how family portraits often reveal not only similar facial features but also similarities in body size, shape and posture? Just as you inherit your skin, eye and hair colour, you inherit your body type. You inherit shapes and sizes of bones and muscles and your capacity for range of motion. It is likely that you inherit a propensity for a certain posture as well. Any of the postures described in this book could be hereditary, yet there are many additional causes for malalignment—injury, for example. This book does not expand on causes because these are numerous and varied. Nevertheless, to give you a flavour of the breadth of possible causal factors, here are examples of some things that may cause malalignment:

- Protracted scapulae may result from overtraining the muscles responsible for protraction, as might be the case in boxing. Or the condition might result from habitual slumped posture as when sitting at a desk. Unilateral protraction could result from holding the bow in archery or might be observed in people whose job or hobby involves repeated flexion of the shoulder, a movement that requires scapular protraction.

- The genu varum knee posture may be the consequence of bowing of the tibia due to mineral deficiency during growth. Or it may be due to osteoarthritis in the knee joint, causing distortion of joint surfaces. Or it could result from overstretching of the lateral collateral ligament due to injury. Or it may develop in response to excessive pronation at the foot and ankle.

- An anteriorly tilted pelvis may be the result of prolonged, repeated overuse of the iliopsoas muscle, pulling the lumbar vertebrae anteriorly. Or it may be the consequence of hypermobility of joints in the lumbar spine. It is frequently observed in the late stages of pregnancy and in people with distended abdomens.

- An increased kyphotic spine may be the result of maintaining a prolonged kyphotic posture, for example as the result of many hours spent on a computer. Or it may be the result of a vertebral fracture resulting in wedging of the thoracic vertebrae, as sometimes occurs with osteoporosis.

- The forward-head posture may result from repeated craning of the head when viewing a computer screen or concentrating on a hobby such as needlework, model making or illustrating. Carrying a heavy backpack intensifies this posture (Chansirinukor et al. 2001).

- Pes planus may be hereditary due to increased weight gain or laxity of ligaments of the foot. It may be associated with an underlying condition, such as Down's syndrome (Dehghani et al. 2012).

- Rotation of the head may be due to maintaining a static head posture to one side, as when watching television. Or it may be due to repeated unilateral rotation, as when looking over the shoulder to reverse a vehicle. Or it may be due to avoidance of neck movement to one side for fear of pain. Or it may be associated with spasm of the cervical rotator muscles.

Bloomfield and colleagues (1994) note a strong relationship between posture and body type (somatotype); the spine is most affected in ectomorphs and the lower limbs are most affected in endomorphs, as summarized in table 1.1.

It would be useful to know whether regular participation in sport causes postural malalignments. Any sport that predominantly uses a muscle or muscle group found to be shortened in a particular posture is likely to perpetuate or worsen that posture. As examples, an exaggerated thoracic kyphosis may be perpetuated by participation in rowing. Rotation of the thorax or tibial torsion might be perpetuated by golf. Genu varum or valgum might be perpetuated by sports involving impact activities such as running or heavy loading of the lower limbs as in weightlifting. Unilateral protraction of the scapulae may be perpetuated by archery or shooting. It seems obvious that sports that use one side of the body more than the other may result in postural imbalance. Hurling, tennis and rowing are such examples and are associated with a high incidence

Table 1.1 Postures Associated With Body Types

Somatotype	Associated posture problems
Ectomorph	Forward head Abducted (protracted) scapulae Increased thoracic kyphosis Increased lumbar lordosis Scoliosis
Endomorph	Genu valgus Pes planus Pes valgus
Mesomorph	Generally free from postural defects but may develop minor problems with age, especially with increased body weight

of scoliosis, asymmetric shoulders and asymmetric back (Watson 1997). Female dragon boat rowers have higher levels of lordosis, lumbar scoliosis and uneven shoulders compared to controls (Pourbehzadi et al. 2012). Although anthropometric measurements are commonly taken to compare sporting and non-sporting individuals, these tend to include items such as proportionality and the importance of limb and body lever lengths rather than the postures described in this book. Studies of athletes focus on physiological—rather than anatomical—profiles, because there is obviously great interest in determining what components make for a great athlete and whether those components can be enhanced. A typical example is a study by Chin and colleagues (1995), which examined elite Asian squash players. Data were collected for pulmonary function, cardiorespiratory fitness, sport-specific fitness, aerobic power, flexibility and muscular strength. Anthropometric data were obtained for height, weight and percentage of body fat. There was no assessment of posture.

By contrast, studies that examine young athletes often include an analysis of posture. A report by Grabara (2012) found that 11- to 14-year-old boys who trained in football three to five times a week had more flattened lumbar lordosis than their untrained peers, whereas Hennessy and Watson (1993) found adult players (including participants from rugby, hurling and Gaelic football) had a *greater* degree of lumbar lordosis. Hennessy and Watson were examining athletes who had sustained hamstring injuries, and this could account for the difference in findings. The authors concluded that certain sports and training methods may exacerbate pre-existing postural defects and predispose a player to injury. They postulated that kicking, straight-leg raising or straight-leg sit-ups used the iliopsoas muscle; this in turn pulled the lumbar spine anteriorly into greater lordosis, the posture they observed in their players. Despite a more malleable spine, repeated use of iliopsoas (as is common in football) did not result in increased lordosis in Grabara's young participants. There may be more data available regarding the posture of young athletes, but for obvious reasons, this cannot be assumed to also describe the posture in adult athletes performing the same sport.

There has been much interest in the posture of the shoulders of athletes, perhaps due to high rates of injury to this part of the body. The shoulders of a healthy athlete have significantly increased upward rotation combined with retraction of the scapulae during humeral elevation compared with the shoulders of non-throwing athletes (Forthomme et al. 2008). This relates to the scapular posture observed at rest: In overhead athletes the dominant shoulder is often positioned lower than the non-dominant shoulder, perhaps due to stretching of ligaments and joint capsules repetitively in a forceful manner (Oyama et al. 2008); the medial border may be more prominent, perhaps due to tightness in the pectoralis minor.

Bloomfield and colleagues (1994) have identified postures that appear to be characteristic of high-performing athletes, based on observation by coaches (table 1.2). It is not clear whether these postures develop as a result of participation in that sport or whether an athlete already had that particular postural characteristic. Bloomfield and colleagues suggest that postures observed in high-performing athletes may be advantageous to that sport and should not be modified but accentuated. Here are examples:

Table 1.2   Postures Observed in and Recommended for High-Performing Athletes

Sport	Posture-related observations and recommendations
Boxing	There is a tendency for round shoulders due to training. (It is not clear whether the authors use the term to mean protracted [abducted] scapulae or internally rotated humeri, or both.)
Contact field sports: Rugby codes Australian football American football	■ Moderate lumbar and thoracic spinal curves are preferable to a non-rigid, non-upright spine. ■ Inverted feet may be advantageous. ■ Anterior pelvic tilt and protruding buttocks may be advantageous. ■ Genu recurvatum is disadvantageous.
Court sports: Basketball Netball Volleyball	■ Inverted feet may be advantageous. ■ Anterior pelvic tilt and protruding buttocks and reasonable thoracic and lumbar curves are needed rather than flattened curves.
Cycling	■ A slightly more rounded back is common to this group of athletes, probably due more to training than to self-selection for success in this sport. ■ Heavy power training may account for enlarged thighs and buttocks.
Gymnastics	■ Female gymnasts with increased lumbar lordosis and anterior pelvic tilt are able to hyperextend the spine more easily than flatter-backed gymnasts. ■ Larger buttocks give gymnasts the advantage of being able to spring more effectively in floor exercises than gymnasts with flat buttocks.
Hurdling	■ A successful hurdler may be tall with anterior pelvic tilt and protruding buttocks.
Jumping	■ Posture of jumping athletes is characterized by an anterior pelvic tilt and protruding buttocks.
Martial arts: Judo Wrestling	■ Inverted feet may be advantageous. ■ Accentuated spinal curves may be advantageous because of enhanced trunk mobility.

(continued)

Table 1.2   *(continued)*

Sport	Posture-related observations and recommendations
Mobile field sports: Field hockey Soccer Lacrosse	■ These athletes vary posturally, and no one posture identified as being advantageous. ■ Inverted feet may be advantageous when the athlete has a limited territory to cover. ■ Anterior pelvic tilt and protruding buttocks may be advantageous where the field position requires high speed over a considerable distance. ■ Moderate lumbar and thoracic spinal curves are preferable to a non-rigid, non-upright spine because players may spend some time in slight spinal flexion during a game. ■ Genu recurvatum is disadvantageous.
Racquet sports: Badminton Racquetball Squash Tennis	■ Inverted feet are advantageous. ■ Compensatory training is required for retaining muscle balance, without which unilateral imbalance and possibly scoliosis would develop due to predominance of one side of the body.
Rowing, canoeing	These athletes have more rounded backs plus a tendency for round shoulders, probably due more to training than to self-selection for success in the sport. (It is not clear whether the authors use the term *round shoulders* to mean protracted [abducted] scapulae or internally rotated humeri, or both.)
Running: middle distance	The shapes of the lumbar spine and buttocks fall between those found in long-distance running and sprinting: 'As the races get longer, the protruding buttock characteristic disappears' (p. 105).
Running: long distance	These athletes have relatively flat buttocks and lumbar spines compared with sprinters.
Running: sprinting	Anterior pelvic tilt and protruding buttocks enhance sprinting.
Throwing	This group varies posturally, and no one posture is identified as being advantageous.
Weightlifting	This group varies posturally, and no one posture is identified as being advantageous.
Set field sports: Baseball Cricket Golf	This group of varies posturally, and no one posture is identified as being advantageous.
Swimming and water polo	■ Swimmers with sloping shoulders have greater shoulder flexion and extension than square-shouldered swimmers, who tend to have larger scapulae and longer clavicles. ■ Swimmers with everted feet are well suited to the leg movements of the breaststroke, whereas swimmers with inward-pointing feet are best suited to leg movements used in the backstroke, freestyle and butterfly. ■ Knee hyperextension may be prevalent in some swimmers, and it has been postulated that this is the result of overstretching of the cruciate ligaments due to repetitive kicking. This posture allows a greater range of anterior and posterior motion at the knee, but it is not clear whether genu recurvatum is advantageous to swimmers.

Data reported by Bloomfield et al. (1994).

- Those with inverted feet have an advantage when running distances of 15 to 20 meters because this posture promotes short, rapid steps, theoretically because tibial torsion shortens the hamstrings, limiting a wider step. There is greater ground contact whilst moving, which might improve dynamic balance.

- An anterior pelvic tilt and protruding buttocks provide an advantage in the extension phase of the running cycle and may therefore be advantageous for players who require sudden bursts of speed.

- Accentuated spinal curves may be advantageous when the sport requires increased trunk mobility.

- Genu recurvatum is disadvantageous to sports requiring twisting and turning running movements as this posture provides reduced knee stability.

Their observations and suggestions raise questions regarding whether to attempt postural correction when working with sport participants.

With the exception of the shoulders of throwing athletes, it is difficult to comment on whether regular participation in any particular sport causes postural malalignments. Much more information is needed regarding the effect of sport on posture, and further studies are required in order to expand on the observations and recommendations put forward by Bloomfield and colleagues (1994).

Consequences of Malalignment

Have you ever seen an image representing a standard or ideal postural alignment, a person standing erect with perfect symmetry? Images such as this are commonly used to illustrate postures in which body parts are least stressed; they are often used as a posture to which we should aspire for aesthetic reasons. Yet the importance of posture may have changed since Victorian times. An aesthetically pleasing posture may be inherent to activities such as dressage or ballet, but few people today strive for good deportment. The well-being of children is as important now as ever, yet teachers are less likely to instruct pupils to sit up straight; and if teachers do tell pupils to sit up straight, it might be a means of retaining attention rather than an attempt to improve posture. Nevertheless, from an anatomical standpoint there are good reasons to consider changing body postures that vary significantly from this ideal. Let's take some aspects of the body and consider the consequences of malalignment to each. As with most of the postures described in this book, the consequences of prolonged alteration in posture to a particular region can only be postulated. In addition to the material provided here, each of the 30 postures in chapters 3 to 10 includes a Consequences section in which you can learn more about the consequences of malalignment to that specific posture.

Bones

When weight-bearing long bones develop with greater curvature than normal, the normal stresses and strains acting on them change. Looking at figure 1.1 consider the tibia of this person's right leg. Compressive forces increase on the concave side of the tibia, whereas tensile forces increase on the convex side. In this example the increased compression is not just on the medial side of the tibia but is also on the anterior aspect (the concave regions of the bone in this example), and the increased strain is not only on the lateral side but also on the posterior of the tibia (the convex regions of the bone). This is because in this person the tibia is bowed not only laterally (figure 1.1a) but also posteriorly (figure 1.1b). If you are not sure that you can see this, take a pen and, using figure 1.1a, trace a line down the centre of the person's right leg, bisecting it longitudinally from the thigh. Notice how your line curves outwards, towards the margin of this book, as you attempt to bisect the calf. The weight of this person is not transmitted optimally through his tibia, nor is the force that is

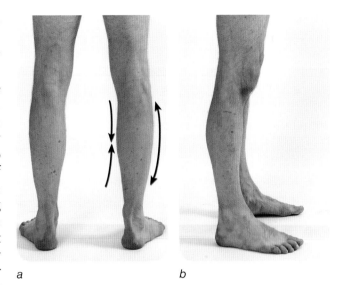

a   b

Figure 1.1   Tibia in this person is both laterally and posteriorly bowed, as shown in posterior (a) and lateral (b) views. Arrows indicate that compressive forces are increased on the concave side of the bone, while tensile forces are increased on the convex side of the bone.

transmitted up through his leg when his feet strike the ground in walking. Because bones are living structures capable of deformation, suboptimal weight bearing through a long bone in this manner could lead to further deformation and therefore a less pleasing appearance for the person. But as stated at the outset, this book is not about changing posture for aesthetic reasons. Why should we bother with a bowed tibia, anatomically speaking? One reason is that a long bone shaped in this manner has reduced load-bearing capabilities and increased risk of injury through, for example, stress fractures. Bowing in a long bone also leads to a change in the immediate joints associated with the bone, in this case the knee (tibiofemoral, patellofemoral and tibiofibular joints), ankle and possibly even joints more remote from this, such as the hip and sacroiliac joint. Overall, the consequence of malalignment is that the bone itself and joints associated with it will not function optimally. The result could be pain in the bone, joints or associated muscles.

Muscles

In the ideal posture, there is minimal strain on soft tissues. If the body is aligned in such a way that muscles remain either actively or passively shortened, they will adapt to their new position and there will be a decrease in the number of sarcomeres from their structure (Heslinga et al. 1995), a decrease in the length of sarcomeres (Spector et al. 1982) and a decrease in the length of tendons (Herbert and Balnave 1993). This is known as adaptive shortening and may mean that the muscle is less able to generate power. When muscles shorten, they hold joints together *more* tightly so there may be a decrease in the range of motion in that joint. Conversely, muscles that remain in a lengthened position add sarcomeres to their length and may weaken. This is known as stretch weakness. When muscles lengthen, they hold joints together *less* tightly. There may be an increased range of motion in that joint. Joints that are too stiff or too mobile could be more easily injured than joints functioning normally.

Anyone who has ever had to maintain a static posture for long will know that muscles quickly develop tension and, if the position is prolonged, it can cause pain. Over time, trigger points may develop, and in chronic cases pain may persist despite a change in body position. The increase in muscle tone may at first be localized to the part of the body that is out of alignment, but as other muscles start to accommodate this dysfunction, the problem spreads. Muscles may fatigue more quickly—first locally, where they cross the affected joint, then distally—and eventually there may be global pain, often in regions distal to the initial site of dysfunction. In severe cases, function is impaired. For example, balance may deteriorate. Mechanical stress perpetuates trigger points; the most common source of this stress is asymmetry and skeletal disproportion (Travell and Simons 1999).

So, these could be the overall effects of malalignment for muscles:

- Increased likelihood of muscle weakness (due to shortening or lengthening of muscles)
- An increase or a decrease in range of motion in a joint
- Possible increase in the likelihood of injury to a joint
- Pain in the affected muscle and in muscles forced to compensate for dysfunction
- Impaired function

Joints

When a joint is not aligned, it also incurs increased stress. Observe the crease on the back of the neck of the person in figure 1.2. What do you think might happen to her cervical joints if she were to maintain this neck position for an hour? What if she maintained this posture all day, whilst performing a desk-based job, for example? Would that give rise to neck pain? What might be the consequences if she maintained the posture all day, every day, for a week? You might expect more frequent neck pain or pain of greater intensity or duration. What if this were the client's normal posture, one that she had inadvertently maintained over many years? Is it reasonable to postulate that in addition to neck pain, there could be a decrease in synovial fluid in cervical joints and a decrease in range of motion at the neck as the joint capsules of cervical vertebrae adhere to local connective tissues? Could the long-term consequences be degeneration of cartilage and early degeneration in the joint? Degeneration would then impinge nerves, resulting in neck, shoulder, back and arm pain.

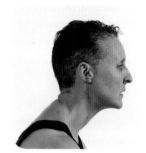

Figure 1.2 Example of a forward head posture.

Ligaments

When a ligament is kept in a lengthened position, it may creep, becoming longer. Longer ligaments provide less stability for the part of the joint that they cross. There may be an increase in range in that joint and even hyperextension of the joint. In figure 1.2, the anterior longitudinal ligament in the cervical region may be lengthened and the posterior longitudinal ligament shortened. This could impair the function of these important structures. Figure 1.3 shows a client with eversion of the ankles. There is increased compressive stress on the lateral side of the ankle and increased tensile stress on the medial side of the ankle. The medial collateral ligaments of the ankle have been overstretched over time, making this person prone to eversion injury (e.g., sprain to the deltoid ligament). Change in the length of a ligament may be minimal, yet if prolonged it will lead to altered biomechanics of that joint and of the joints above and below it. Injury to a

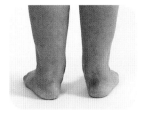

Figure 1.3 Altered ankle alignment affecting ligaments of the ankle.

ligament can also lead to postural change. Anterior cruciate ligament (ACL) rupture, for example, increases the risk of knee osteoarthritis, which is associated with genu valgum and varum postures. It is not known whether rupture of an important ligament such as the ACL predisposes a person to the development of genu valgum or varum postures.

Lengthening of ligaments means not only is that particular joint less stable, but also the joints above and below it are too, because these joints become subject to additional stresses and strains. Therefore, someone with lengthened ligaments in the knee is at greater risk of hip and ankle injuries on the affected side, and someone with lengthened ligaments in the elbow is at greater risk of shoulder and wrist injuries on the affected side. Ligaments contain nerve endings that are important for reflex and proprioceptive function. Constant compression or tensioning of ligaments—rather than the normal varying of compression or tension as occurs during movement or weight bearing—may adversely affect function of nerve endings.

Other Soft Tissues

As with bones, joints, muscles and ligaments, a posture that results in increased compressive or tensile forces on soft tissues such as blood vessels, lymph vessels, nerves or fascia is likely to adversely affect how those tissues function. Have you observed what skin looks like when a plaster cast has been removed? Compressed beneath the cast, the skin appears pale and lifeless. You can observe this also on removal of an adhesive bandage, even when it has been worn for just a few days. Skin does not respond well to being permanently compressed, albeit lightly. The compression—or traction—of soft tissues within the body is not visible; such a condition may coincide with a prolonged alteration in posture, but these structures are likely to be as affected by malalignment as muscles, tendons and ligaments are.

Perhaps the most significant consequence of mal-alignment is that the 30 postures described in this book are each likely to worsen if not treated. The degree to which they worsen is likely to vary; some postures will worsen to a greater extent than others. For example, a person with a kyphotic posture can become increasingly kyphotic, but a person with a flatfoot posture cannot necessarily get a *more* flattened foot. How quickly a posture worsens is also highly variable. It may worsen within months or over many years, and the progression depends on many factors. Examples are the stage at which the posture is identified, the person's underlying health, the availability of professionals able to provide advice and treatment and the willingness and ability of the client to engage in postural correction activities. Consider two sisters with a familial history of genu valgus, both having noticed that they too have a mild genu valgus posture in one knee. One sister continues to enjoy bootcamp-type exercise involving weightlifting and running and is unconcerned with her knee posture. The other sister seeks advice and learns that neither weightlifting nor running is favourable for the genu valgum posture. Weightlifting places excessive load through the malaligned joint, whilst running involves repeated impact. The second sister explores the many other sporting options available, such as non-impact activities like swimming and cycling and rowing, and uses some of the recommendations set out in this book for management of the genu valgum posture. It seems likely that the sister who engages in activity that is unfavourable to this posture is likely to have a worsening of the posture more quickly than her counterpart.

When a client comes to you for hands-on therapy, postural assessment is important because the advice you can give after early identification of malalignments can help a client to avoid aggravating factors and adopt exercises and treatments that minimise further disruption of the joint. More information on broaching the subject of postural correction is in chapter 2 in the section titled Gaining Rapport and Enhancing Engagement as well as the section in chapter 6 titled What You Can Do as a Therapist.

Who Might Benefit From Postural Correction?

The 30 postures described in *Postural Correction* are not specific to any one population, and many clients are likely to benefit from advice on avoiding or correcting postures that are likely to cause unwanted symptoms. The following list is not exhaustive but provides examples of the kinds of clients who may be susceptible to malalignment and for whom postural correction may be beneficial:

- Elderly people are more likely to present with genu valgum or genu varum when they are in the advanced stages of osteoarthritis. These postures can also be seen in people who have suffered knee injury or where injury or pathology affects the hips or ankles.

- The elderly are frequently observed to have kyphotic thoracic spines. So too are people who sit for prolonged periods or whose occupations involve repeated stooping.

- Many manual workers have asymmetric postures. For example, in the days when refuse bins were carried and emptied manually, refuse collectors portrayed lateral flexion of the spine as they repeatedly contracted muscles on one side in order to pick up and transport a dustbin. Whether such a working posture develops into true postural change is unknown but provides a good example of an activity that could lead to postural imbalance. Lateral flexion of the spine can also be observed in anyone who repeatedly carries a heavy bag on one side of the body. Vehicle-based camera crews filming sporting events have to look upwards to television screens for long periods, and at rest they may be observed to have hyperextension of the cervical spine. This is also common in linesmen employed to maintain overhead electrical cables, a job that necessitates climbing telegraph poles or using mobile elevated platforms whilst looking upwards. People with certain medical conditions are predisposed to malalignment. For example, hypermobile people lack stability in their joints and are likely to suffer increased cervical lordosis due to spondylolisthesis. Scoliosis is seen in 30% to 50% of people with Ehlers-Danlos syndrome hypermobility type; 23.7% have thoracic kyphosis and 43% to 55% have acquired flatfoot, and genu valgum often results from this foot posture (Tinkle 2008). In a study of 30 female teenagers with Down's syndrome,

Dehghani and colleagues (2012) report the following percentages relating to specific postures: flatfoot (96%), genu valgum (83%), increased lumbar lordosis (63%), torticollis (lateral neck flexion) (60%), genu recurvatum (43%), kyphosis (10%), scoliosis (6%) and genu varum (3%).

- People who sustain injury to a joint may undergo a change in the posture of that joint, something that may be exacerbated through weight bearing. People who sustain injury during childhood sometimes develop marked asymmetrical postures in the lower limb and spine as they avoided bearing weight on the injured side. In some cases they never develop weight bearing equally through both lower limbs and show an unconscious preference for the uninjured side, despite having recovered many years previously from the initial injury.

- Non-symmetrical cervical postures may be observed in some people after whiplash injury.

- Pregnant women often appear to have increased lordotic lumbar spines, in which the spine is pulled forward due to the additional weight carried anteriorly.

- In addition to the postures described by Bloomfield and colleagues, in table 1.2 you can observe specific postures in sportspeople:
  - The upper fibres of the trapezius muscles in tennis players tend to hypertrophy on the dominant side due to repeated elevation of the batting arm above shoulder height. The scapula on the dominant side of asymptomatic tennis players has been found to be more protracted than the scapula on the non-dominant side, and this asymmetry may be normal for this group of sportspeople (Oyama et al. 2008).
  - Golfers may develop postures associated with rotation not just in the back and hips but at the knees and feet also.
  - Boxers may have elbows that are flexed at rest due to hypertrophy and shortening of the elbow flexor muscles.
  - Practitioners of wing chun kung fu frequently demonstrate internal rotation of both the hips and shoulders. This is because of the stance adopted for practicing many of the chi saus, the repetitive arm movements inherent to this form of martial art.
- Postural problems also develop in association with immobility:
  - People who work at desks often display internal rotation of the shoulders and thoracic kyphosis due to prolonged sitting postures.
  - People who use wheelchairs or who spend many hours sitting or driving as part of their occupation may develop postures associated with hip and knee flexion.

Contraindications to and Cautions for Postural Correction

Most of the techniques described in *Postural Correction* are suitable for most people. However, care is required when attempting to help some people to correct posture using the techniques described in this book. Where caution is needed, or where a technique is specifically contraindicated, this is noted in the information in each relevant section.

The cautions and contraindication are comprehensive but not exhaustive. As a qualified practitioner you should follow the guidelines set out by your governing body for the delivery of the therapies in which you are qualified and insured to practice. If you are ever in doubt, choose an alternative method of treatment you know to be appropriate.

When Care Is Needed

- Addressing posture in clients likely to have osteoporosis (e.g., elderly or anorexic clients or clients *formerly* anorexic or bulimic). If you know or suspect your client has osteoporosis, you should avoid applying all but the lightest pressure to bones. When applying stretches, some degree of tension is needed, and this often places pressure on bones and joints. Avoid stretching.

- Working with clients who have adopted postures in response to ongoing painful conditions. Avoid trying to correct posture in a client who is leaning to one side, for example, to avoid pain in the back. First address underlying causes of pain.

- Working with clients whose postures are protective in nature and adopted consciously or unconsciously in response to emotional sensitivity (e.g., fear, anxiety, shyness, depression). Changing from a closed to an open posture, from a kyphotic to a more upright extended spinal posture, for example, can have profound effects on emotion. In such cases it is often helpful to attempt small changes, giving your client the opportunity to acclimatize over the course of a week or several weeks, before continuing treatment.

- Working with hypermobile clients. Adults with hypermobility have flexibility at the expense of strength. These clients have extra laxity in their soft tissues, and the focus of your treatment should be to shorten tissues, not to lengthen them. In some cases localized areas of tension can be treated; remember, though, where a client has true hypermobility syndrome, it is not just the joints that are affected. There may be weakness in skin and blood vessels also. You will need to refer such clients to specialists.

- Addressing posture in clients whose postures result from excessively high muscle tone. Specialist advice is often needed when working with such clients. Tone may be the result of the underlying condition (e.g., spasticity in the elbow flexors associated with cerebral palsy or after a stroke) or could be a consequence of medication, in which case attempting to decrease tone in order to improve posture could be futile.

- Addressing posture in clients whose postures result from low tone. Tone may be the result of the underlying condition (e.g., a dropped shoulder after stroke or dropped foot after tibial nerve injury), in which case attempting to increase tone in order to improve posture may be ineffective.

- Treating a pregnant client or within 12 months postnatally. Pregnancy alters posture temporarily, and whilst it is preferable to address postural concerns postnatally, relaxin may be present in the body for many months after birthing. This is responsible for increasing pliability of soft tissues, so take care not to overstretch the soft tissues.

- Working with elderly clients. Aging brings about a decrease in pliability in soft tissues and, in some cases, weakening of bones. Take extra care when treating these clients.

- Working with children. Although children and adolescents benefit from postural correction, this requires specialist intervention and is beyond the scope of this book. This is because certain postures that are considered disadvantageous in adults are normal in growing children.

CONTRAINDICATIONS

- Acute conditions at the site of treatment or that may be affected by treatment to another part of the body
- Inflammatory conditions
- Haematoma
- Vascular disorders of the vertebral artery
- Osteoporosis and patients at risk of fracture
- Malignancy
- Bone or joint limitation due to fusion (pathological or surgical)
- Acute thrombus or embolism
- Where a muscle contributes to stability of a joint and lengthening it would impair that stability
- Where the treatment may compromise the healing process of any condition (e.g., in stressing a not-yet-healed scar or recent burn)
- When the treatment could reverse or impair the benefit of another treatment
- When treating a patient for whom it is not known whether the technique will be beneficial and where medical permission has not been granted
- Where the application causes pain

- Additionally, care is needed when treating clients with these conditions:
  - Unable to provide feedback
  - Fragile skin
  - At high risk of infection through touch
  - Nervous, anxious, or emotional about physical touch
  - After long-term use of steroids
  - Balance problems
  - Unable to safely follow instructions

As with any treatment, you should discuss your intentions with your client and gain consent before proceeding. More information about treatment techniques is in chapter 2.

Closing Remarks

This chapter contains examples of the causes of postural malalignment, and you have learnt that malalignment could result in a change in the shape of a bone, muscle, joint or body part and a change in overall posture. Malalignment can also impair function in a body part and cause pain or other symptoms in that part or even in parts remote from the one in question. The chapter includes examples of clients who may be predisposed to postural problems and examples of clients who may benefit from postural correction. Most people can receive postural correction, but there are some precautions to consider. In some cases, correction is specifically contraindicated.

Changing Posture

Learning Outcomes

After reading this chapter, you should be able to do the following:

- List five steps to postural correction.
- Give examples of techniques that may be used in each of these steps.
- Describe why the identification of causal factors is so important for the correction of posture and why client-led correction may have a greater impact than corrective techniques used by a therapist.
- Give the rationale for the use of stretching, massage, strengthening, deactivation of trigger points and taping in postural correction.
- Give examples of general guidelines for postural correction.
- Give examples of guidelines specific to the use of stretching, massage, strengthening, deactivation of trigger points and taping, along with any cautions and contraindications.
- Give examples of when referral to another practitioner may be warranted.

This chapter presents guidelines for techniques used in correcting posture. The ideas are for use when working with adults, and it is assumed that you are attempting to correct an established posture, not what is present post-operatively or immediately after trauma. For example, a patient may present with a knee flexion deformity due to a torn hamstring or after knee surgery; in each case you would follow the normal rehabilitative procedures (i.e., reducing the inflammatory stage with rest, ice, compression and elevation) before moving on to gentle mobilization of soft tissues in order to reduce the likelihood of scar formation. You would not attempt to use the corrective techniques described in this book in the early stages of repair and rehabilitation. It is assumed that, as a therapy or exercise professional, you have the skills to decide at which point it is safe to start corrective treatment.

The training of bodyworkers, whether as massage therapists, physiotherapists, sport therapists, osteopaths or chiropractors, involves giving and receiving assessments as well as hands-on treatments. You are probably accustomed to being observed and handled by classmates. Most therapists engage in continuing professional development, and most become relaxed with learning new techniques in the presence of strangers (i.e., therapists they may never have met). Seeing so many body types, you become comfortable with the body and may even become blasé about your own body. You accept that imperfection is commonplace and that all humans are uniquely perfect. However, it does not hurt to keep in mind that many of the clients you treat will not have had these experiences and may be far less comfortable in being physically assessed or receiving hands-on treatment than you are. Sensitivity is essential when treating any client for postural correction. If the posture is pronounced, the client may not feel comfortable with the appearance of her body. Where it is mild, it is important to avoid emotive comments. Most therapists are extremely careful in their use of words when speaking with clients. Even common words—such as *twisted*, *rotated*, *curved* or *bent*—when used to describe the spine or a joint can leave a client feeling alarmed. Avoid words such as *malaligned* and *abnormal* entirely.

In conveying the shape of posture to a client who has come to you for advice on postural correction, one suggestion is to use less emotive words, such as *asymmetrical,* or to say there is slight deviation. Obviously you cannot describe a very pronounced posture in this way. A second suggestion is to show your client his posture in a mirror or photograph and ask him how he would describe it. You could continue to use any words or phrases the client uses in further discussions. How you approach the discussion regarding treatment of posture stems entirely from the information gathered during the initial consultation, the descriptions your client provides to describe his posture, his descriptions of past treatment, and the rapport you develop at this crucial stage of the client–therapist relationship.

Determining the Start of Postural Correction

When treatment for postural correction should begin is a difficult question to answer. In some cases a client may approach you specifically requesting advice on postural change (as in some of the examples provided later in this chapter). However, it is more common to observe postural imbalance on a client's initial visit when you conduct your initial assessment. If you believe that correction of posture will alleviate symptoms, then it is important to build postural correction into the treatment plan as soon as possible. Whether a change in a joint prevents permanent damage is not known and depends on the degree to which that body part is misaligned, the stage of underlying pathology (if there is one), factors perpetuating the malalignment (such as sporting activity) and the skills you have at your disposal to make the necessary changes. Combined with this is the client's willingness to participate in postural change.

You learnt in chapter 1 that malalignment can have adverse effects on bones, joints, ligaments and other structures at a local level. It may even lead to poor healing and pathological changes (Troyanovich et al. 1998). A good argument for minimizing the likelihood of this happening is by attempting to correct posture. Yet, when changes are made to any one body part, they affect the posture of other body parts. For example, in the lower limb, abnormal posture in a joint of the foot, ankle, knee or hip affects how load is transferred throughout the entire limb. Hypo- or hypermobility at the foot and ankle reduces the ability of the foot to act as a shock absorber and torque convertor, so the patient is less able to adapt to the terrain and no longer has a rigid lever to push off from (Donatelli 1987). To compensate for deformity, the motion of adjacent joints is altered, gait pattern may change and muscles are likely to fatigue as they work harder to resist abnormal loads and maintain joint position (Fawdington et al. 2013). The segmental nature of the body means that altering one body part affects other segments in a way that may be positive or negative, and the affected segments will themselves impact on additional segments. Hypomobile joints may force adjacent joints to compensate, becoming hypermobile to enable a full range of motion (Hertling and Kessler 2006). Failing to address all of the affected segments may reduce the impact of an intervention. There is disagreement about which part of the body most affects the posture of other parts. What seems clear is that an adjustment to any one part has significant—though not necessarily immediate—impact on the entire body.

One of the principles underlying postural correction is the correct identification of what Lee (2013) calls a primary driver. This is the anatomical component of posture most likely to contribute to the maintenance of that posture. In all postures there are multiple contributing anatomical factors, and your task is to identify what to alter to bring about the most significant change. Identification of the primary driver can be difficult for many reasons. In the lower limb, for example, compensatory motions do not occur in a predictable manner (Gross 1995). Assessing joints is a specialized skill and can be time consuming, even for experienced practitioners. One study concluded that key examinations used in assessing foot function were unreliable and that using such assessments to differentiate between normal and pathological foot function were not valid (Jarvis et al. 2012), despite the assessments carried out by podiatrists with at least five years of experience. Also, there is disagreement about which parts of the body are most significant in causing or contributing to unfavourable postures. Podiatrists are likely to be aware that orthotics for the control of supination or pronation, for example, can have a profound effect on pain and dysfunction in the entire lower limb (Donatelli 1987) and might argue that if foot posture is abnormal, it will affect not only the lower limb but the pelvis and right up through the spine to the thorax and head. Some therapists argue that postural imbalance begins at the opposite end of the body; that the weight of the head is significant in initiating dysfunction in the cervical, thoracic and eventually lumbar spine; and that the spine is altered to accommodate changes in head position. Others might argue that the correct position of the pelvis, being the anchor between the upper and lower body, is crucial to the correction of posture elsewhere.

You might have discovered from your own practice that certain postures coincide with one another? For example, the forward head posture coincides with kyphosis in the thorax; an anterior pelvic tilt often coincides with hyperextension at the knee; lateral tilt of the head and neck correspond with an elevated shoulder; rotation of the pelvis corresponds with torsion of the tibia. There is little evidence that clarifies whether one posture causes another. Even once you have identified the joint you believe to be the most significant contributing component to the posture you wish to change, you may not know what has given rise to the joint problem itself. Where a patient with normal knee alignment suffers a serious knee injury, after which the knee is observed to be malaligned, the injury is the cause of the malalignment. However, it is more difficult to attribute malalignment to a particular factor where change is insidious: Genu varum knee posture could develop as the result of injury, because of the gradual weakening of ligaments due to disease, as the result of underlying pathology such as hypermobility, because of a bowing of the tibia, because the client is in a demographic prone to genu varum, or because the client injured the ankle on the other leg as a child and bore weight excessively through the genu varum knee for many years. As Hertling and Kessler (2006) state, there is no single cause of joint dysfunction. Fortunately, massage therapists, exercise professionals and students of physiotherapy, chiropractic and osteopathy for whom this book is intended are not expected to be able to diagnose complex biomechanical irregularities. They are, however, able to identify general postural imbalance and shortened soft tissues. Use this book as a starting point for your exploration into postural correction, and bear in mind that the techniques described in this chapter are not exhaustive; they are selected on the grounds of those most likely to fall within your remit and because they are likely to be safe for use with most clients.

Five Steps to Postural Correction

The following five steps are offered as a means of correcting posture, and table 2.1 provides examples of techniques that might help you achieve each step. These techniques are later described in more detail along with the rationale for their use and guidelines for implementation.

The first step is to identify contributing factors to this posture and eliminate or reduce those factors. Whether the posture has arisen for an obvious reason such as an injury or surgery or whether it developed insidiously is likely to come to light during your initial assessment when you ask your client to provide medical history. A full-body postural assessment will provide additional information from which you may choose to explore segments of the body in more detail using palpation and movement tests. If you are not certain how to assess posture, see *Postural Assessment* (Johnson 2012). Subjective feedback concerning occupation and recreational and sporting activity is essential in establishing extrinsic factors likely to affect a client's posture.

Steps 2 and 3 are two sides of the same coin. Step 2 is to increase the range of motion in hypomobile segments. Correcting the alignment of a joint involves both increasing range of motion in hypomobile joints and decreasing range of motion in hypermobile joints. Mobility of joints may be improved by lengthening shortened soft tissues specific to that joint; using techniques such as active or passive stretching, traction, and massage; and deactivating trigger points. Techniques such as myofascial release are helpful because they facilitate a general unwinding in the body.

Step 3 is to decrease movement in hypermobile segments. Decreasing movement in a hypermobile joint helps stabilize that joint. You might achieve this by shortening the tissues that are lengthened through the use of strengthening exercises. Taping and bracing may also be used to limit joint mobility.

Once you decrease movement in hypermobile segments, maintaining normal joint position is step 4. One of the key techniques in maintaining a realigned joint is avoiding perpetuating factors, where possible. For example, if the joint in question is the knee, you should advise the client to avoid sitting on the foot and ankle if she reports it as a habit, because sitting on the foot in this way places uneven stress through the knee joint even though there is no weight bearing through the knee itself in this position.

Step 5 is to re-educate movement patterns. Joints that have been malaligned have a tendency to stay that way unless the neural mechanisms responsible for joint position and movement are re-educated to acknowledge the improved joint position. This is a specialized field of therapy that requires movement to be controlled under the guidance of a therapist who can intervene to make minor adjustments in the hope that this will eventually bring about 'remembering' the original, more correct joint position.

Table 2.1 Techniques That Support Postural Correction

Step	Example of technique used
Step 1: Identify contributing factors to the posture and eliminate or reduce them.	Take a medical history and note subjective feedback from the client. Is there an underlying pathology (e.g., arthritis, recent injury, hypermobility, ankylosing spondylitis)? Does the client mention anything that might contribute to the postural problem? For example, sleeping in the prone position may aggravate an increased lumbar lordosis, letting the knees lock out (hyperextend) when standing will aggravate genu recurvatum; always carrying a heavy bag on the same shoulder will likely maintain elevation of that shoulder.
	Gross, full-body postural assessment. For example, does the client have a particular stance that may aggravate a posture? Is there evidence of previous injury that might account for the posture? Does the client use a walking aid?
	Localized assessment of joints and tissues using palpation and assessment of joint range. What do muscle length tests reveal?
	Assessment of occupational, sporting or recreational postures. Is there a posture your client maintains for prolonged periods?
Step 2: Increase range of motion in hypomobile joints.	Lengthen shortened soft tissues specific to that joint using techniques such as active or passive stretching, traction, massage, deactivation of trigger points, myofascial release and repositioning.
	Joint mobilization or manipulation.
Step 3: Decrease range of motion in hypermobile joints.	Strengthening lengthened muscles specific to that joint by using simple home exercises or exercises performed under supervision.
	Taping and bracing.
Step 4: Maintain normal joint position.	Avoiding habitually abnormal postures.
	Taping.
	Bracing and supports.
Step 5: Re-educate movement patterns.	Specific techniques used by sport therapists and physiotherapists.

Techniques for Postural Correction

Because this book is in a series aimed primarily, but not solely, at therapists who employ hands-on techniques, the techniques selected are those that fall within the remit of massage therapists and exercise professionals and students of physiotherapy, osteopathy, chiropractic and sport therapy. Joint mobilization and manipulation, the use of specific neural re-education and use of orthotics have been deliberately omitted because these techniques require specialist training that falls outside the remit of readers for whom *Postural Correction* is intended. The techniques in this book are aimed at helping soft tissues to function in a more optimal manner to reduce compressive and tensile forces by lengthening shortened tissues and shortening lengthened tissues. These techniques bring about a more normal alignment of body parts and sustain those positions:

- Identifying and avoiding causal habits
- Stretching
- Massage
- Deactivation of trigger points
- Muscle strengthening
- Taping, bracing and casting

In the world of therapy there has been a move away from passive intervention towards greater emphasis on the self-management of conditions. This is true for postural correction. Either the client or the therapist can use many of the techniques described here and, where possible, emphasis should be on the client's use. The rationale for this is that outcomes tend to be better when clients take more active roles in their rehabilitation. It seems logical also that with your advice, a client will be able to devote more time to the correction of posture and may therefore have a greater impact than you might achieve in one or two treatment sessions that are weeks apart.

Adaptive shortening occurs as the result of a muscle remaining in a shortened position (Heslinga et al. 1995; Spector et al. 1982; Herbert and Balnave 1993). The rationale for stretching, massage and deactivation of trigger points is that they help lengthen shortened tissues and therefore increase mobility of a joint. Some of the claims made for massage are that it may restore extensibility of soft tissues, promote relaxation of muscles, loosen scar tissue, stretch tight muscles and fascia and reduce muscle spasm. Perhaps this is why some therapists believe that 'Stretching massage is invaluable in the corrective treatment of muscle and fascia shortened by longstanding postural faults or immobilization' (Kendall et al. 1993, p. 337).

If tightness in soft tissues is not countered by the opposing muscle, the resting position of the joint changes and the overall result is a restriction in range of motion. The rationale for strengthening is that it helps shorten tissues and therefore helps reduce mobility in a joint. It is used for muscles found to be lengthened in hypermobile joints. It may also help increase extensibility in the opposing muscle group and may therefore be used in the correction of hypomobile joints (e.g., contracting rhomboids to facilitate a stretch in the pectorals).

Taping, bracing and casts are used to maintain correct joint alignment once this has been achieved. In some cases such devices are used to prevent worsening of joint alignment where further advances in treatment are unlikely. The rationale underpinning splinting is to provide a prolonged stretch to maintain or promote change in a body structure (College of Occupational Therapists and Association of Chartered Physiotherapists in Neurology 2015). In an ideal situation devices are used in the short term only. They may be useful as an adjunct to treatment.

The rationale for various treatment techniques is summarized in table 2.2.

Determining the frequency of treatment for postural correction is difficult. As the client examples provided at the end of this chapter demonstrate, the frequency of treatment needs to be tailored to the individual. Unfortunately, we do not have information to support a particular frequency of treatment for particular techniques. For example, we do not know whether treating a client once a week with passive stretching will be more effective, less effective or the same as treating them once a week with massage to lengthen tissues. It seems reasonable that frequent intervention is likely to be effective in correcting posture where postural correction is possible. However, encouraging a client to believe that she needs the input of a therapist for prolonged periods, whether on a regular basis or even infrequently, is questionable ethically. In some cases it may be necessary to set appointments at specific intervals, but in many cases, frequency of appointments will depend on the progress. Initially it is undeniable that the client will

Table 2.2   Treatment Techniques, Rationale and Utility

Technique	Rationale	Used to address
Identification and avoidance of causal habits	Postures adopted on a regular basis perpetuate themselves; by avoiding them, patients facilitate postural change.	Ongoing activities likely to perpetuate and aggravate the posture in question
Stretching (all forms), massage (deep tissue), deactivation of trigger points	All help to lengthen shortened tissues and therefore help increase joint mobility.	Hypomobility in a joint
Myofascial release	Facilitates an overall release in fascia and therefore helps increase joint mobility.	Hypomobility in a joint
Muscle strengthening	Shortens muscles and therefore reduces mobility in a joint.	Hyper- or hypomobility in a joint depending on treatment objective
Taping, bracing, casts	Helps maintain correct joint alignment once it has been achieved, or in some cases prevents worsening of existing joint alignment.	Maintenance of a joint position

require therapeutic intervention in the correction of posture, but the intervention should be weighted towards supporting the activities the client carries out for himself—change in habitual patterns, active engagement in stretching and strengthening of muscles, willingness to adopt a different work posture or to investigate changing the way he swings a golf club, for example. A desirable outcome might be to provide 5 to 10 treatments

GENERAL GUIDELINES FOR POSTURAL CORRECTION

You need to consider guidelines for postural correction before delivering any intervention. In each treatment technique section you will find additional guidelines specific to that treatment.

- It is customary to instruct therapists to use techniques that are evidence based, which involves the explicit and judicious use of current research in making decisions about the care of patients (Sackett 1996). Unfortunately, there is little information on how best to correct posture.
- Tailor any intervention to the specific needs of your client.
- Take baseline measurements in the form of range of motion, photographs or subjective feedback. In a survey of complementary and alternative medicine interventions used by researchers, practitioners and students, 92 outcome measures were identified (Verhoef et al. 2006). These included physical, psychological, social, spiritual, quality of life and holistic measures. Remember that you need to be able to determine whether the treatment you provide—whether by hands-on therapy or through advice—is effective, and to do this you need to decide early on how you will measure effectiveness.
- Consider contraindications and cautions. Most of the techniques described in this book are safe to use with most people. However, you need to consider certain contraindications and cautions when treating certain client groups (see chapter 1).
- Always work within your professional remit and use techniques in which you are trained. If in doubt, follow the guidelines set forth by your governing body.
- Wherever possible, work with your client to set SMART treatment goals: goals that are Specific, Measureable, Achievable, Realistic and Time bound. There is more about goal setting in the section Gaining Rapport and Enhancing Engagement later in this chapter.
- Document all of your interventions and client feedback using both quantitative and qualitative data.
- If you agree that one of the problems resulting from postural imbalance is pain, then it seems reasonable to start with whichever treatment intervention is most likely to reduce pain.
- Reassess posture after intervention.
- Adjust interventions according to outcomes.

initially scheduled close together but gradually occurring further apart so that at the last appointment, you are eventually just checking that all is well and that your client is now on the road to management of his own condition. In all therapeutic interventions the intention is to wean the client off therapy from the earliest possible time, and it is preferable—though not always possible—to avoid reliance on the therapist for treatment from the onset.

It is not known how long it takes to correct posture. Troyanovich and colleagues (1998) have suggested that treatment and prevention of spinal pathologies beyond the resolution of symptoms should involve an aggressive rehabilitation programme of 3 to 6 months but highlights the need for further research. Remodelling of connective tissue occurs over an extended period, and daily stretching may be necessary for maintaining lasting improvement in range of motion (Jacobs and Sciascia 2011); When working with athletes, postural correction requires an intense programme spanning several years (Bloomfield et al. 1994).

Identification and Avoidance of Causal Habits

This is included as a technique because it is so important to the correction of posture. The physiological benefits of postural correction may be short lived if your client returns to those behaviours that were significant in bringing about such posture. Is your client performing some activity in her occupation, sport or recreational activity that contributes to the perpetuation of this posture? In some cases a client may know what these behaviours are. For example, she may have realized that wearing high heels shortens calf muscles because when she wears flat-heeled shoes, she has pain or a stretching sensation in those muscles. In many cases a client may be unaware that a behaviour is aggravating a particular posture. For example, regularly using the same hand to carry a heavy bag or always slinging a rucksack over the same shoulder results in more frequent contraction of levator scapulae muscles on that shoulder than of the other shoulder.

In a random selection of 100 participants, Guimond and Massrieh (2012) found a correlation between a person's demeanour and posture (see table 2.3), supporting the notion that the body shapes itself into various postures depending on the underlying mental and emotional state. Grouping particpants according to the four postures described by Kendall and McCreary (1983), they used a Myers-Briggs Type Indicator to determine characteristics of personality and discovered a relationship between posture type and two aspects of personality: extroversion and introversion. For example, they found that 96% of participants with 'perfect posture' were extrovert and only 4% were introvert, whereas the converse was true for participants with a kyphosis–lordosis

Table 2.3   Four Types of Posture Correlated With Two Aspects of Personality

Posture	Extrovert	Introvert
Ideal	96%	4%
Kyphosis–lordosis	17%	83%
Flatback	42%	58%
Swayback	26%	74%

Data from Guimond and Massrieh 2012.

posture, where only 17% were extrovert and 83% were introvert. This makes for slightly uncomfortable reading. If postural deviations are purely anatomical, manual correction of a joint or joints by either the client or a therapist is a good starting point in minimizing, eradicating or preventing an undesirable posture. There are enough variables to make this challenging. To add the variable of whether your client's personality might be correlated with posture raises many questions. For example, when attempting to correct the kyphosis–lordosis posture of your client, which Guimond and Massrieh found to correlate with the introverted personality type, would you be more successful if your client agreed to behave in a manner normally associated with extroversion? Can personality types be changed from introvert to extrovert, and would this affect posture?

There may, however, be a link between posture and emotion. Consider what happens to your own posture when you feel embarrassed, shy, ashamed, uncertain or withdrawn. Do you flex your spine, lower your head, flex your elbows, bring your hand to your mouth or jaw or hug yourself, making yourself physically smaller? Compare this to how your posture changes when you feel confident, certain and elated. Does your spine straighten, do you raise your head and do you pull back your shoulders? Changing how you feel affects muscle tone and overall posture, so the significance of the part played by your client in helping to correct his own posture—whether via physiological or emotional means—cannot be overemphasized.

Helping Your Client Identify, Eliminate or Reduce Causal Habits

- Use of pertinent questions during the subject stage of your assessment will help you identify factors that contribute to the posture that needs correction. A change in posture may be acute (e.g., an altered upper-limb posture after elbow fracture or altered neck or back posture associated with sudden spasm of a muscle), or it may be insidious (e.g., with progressive arthritis in the knee). Ask your client whether she regularly sustains a particular posture or regularly performs a repetitive action. These are likely to be contributing factors to imbalance in the body.

- Encourage your client to take an active part in the correction of posture.

- Encourage honest feedback. For example, did he do all of the exercises and stretches?

- Avoid overloading a client with too many stretches or exercises; instead, help him to focus on performing one or two correctly.

- Explain that, in some cases, correction can take weeks or months, depending on how long the body part has been out of alignment. In some cases correction may be readily attained, but what is important is *sustained* correction. Expecting gradual progress is probably a more realistic expectation than wanting immediate results.

- If you believe that some aspect of your client's work environment may be contributing to his posture, you may wish to refer him to the occupational health department of his organization, if there is one, or to an ergonomist. Factors affecting work-related musculoskeletal conditions are complex, and interventions require a tailored approach (Panel on Musculoskeletal Disorders and the Workplace Commission on Behavioral and Social Sciences and Education National Research Council and Institute of Medicine 2001). It seems reasonable that postural problems believed to have a work-related component are also likely to be complex and require an individualized approach.

- If your client has a job in which he remains seated at a computer, an ideal situation is for you to visit him and to assess how he is using the computer. Provide advice on basic computer setup and, if possible, follow the guidelines set forth in the appendix: Correct setup for display screen equipment to minimize postural stress in sitting. Give this advice to your client verbally and in printed form. Many sources of information are available for your client to refer to should he fall back into bad habits. Examples are *Working With Display Screen Equipment* (Health & Safety Executive 2013), *How to Sit at a Computer* (American Academy of Orthopaedic Surgeons 2007), *Perfect Posture* (Chartered Society of Physiotherapists 2013) and *Ergonomics Program: The Computer Workstation* (National Institutes of Health 2014).

- Discourage reliance on your intervention in the long term. Hopefully, you will work with your client to help him correct a certain posture, and in doing so he will become aware of poor postural habits. Many professional sources are available for tips on postural correction, such as the American Chiropractic Association (2014). Your client may turn to these for gentle reminders on sitting, standing and sleeping postures in general.

Stretching

Muscles that have become short and weak may restrict the normal range of motion in a joint, preventing realignment. The joint may be held in such a position that active stretches are difficult to achieve. So, do you stretch and lengthen short muscles first, or do you shorten and strengthen long muscles first? It might seem not to matter where you start, whether you stretch out a tight muscle first or you rely on strengthening weakened muscles in the hope that, through reciprocal inhibition, contraction of an agonist will bring about relaxation of its antagonist. However, there is clinical and scientific evidence to support stretching and normalizing of tight muscles before strengthening of weak muscles begins (Chaitow 2001).

Either the client or the therapist can perform stretching of shortened tissues. To facilitate change, an intervention that is performed on a regular basis is likely to be more effective than the same intervention performed less frequently. Therefore, active stretching—that performed only by the client—may be of greater benefit to the correction of posture than passive stretching. The advantages of active stretching are that your client can perform this daily, whereas passive stretching is used during a treatment session, which in many cases may be only once a week. Disadvantages of active stretching are that the client may perform stretches incorrectly or may lose the motivation to perform them at all. Where very specific, localized stretching is required, this may be better performed by a therapist, who can identify and target tissues. In some cases it may be difficult or impossible for a client to target these tissues herself. For example, in the case of thoracic flatback (see chapter 4), a client may have tension in a specific segment of the spine, and flexing the thoracic spine is likely to stretch the paraspinal muscles as a whole rather than the localized area of tissue tension.

Throughout this book are examples of the active stretches traditionally used to lengthen specific muscles, and in many cases these stretch more than one muscle. Stretching also occurs in soft tissues when a client rests. Therefore, specific resting postures may help bring about lengthening in tissues you have identified as being shortened.

The following information sets out guidelines for the use of active and passive stretching, including specialized forms of stretching such as traction, soft tissue release and muscle energy technique. The recommendations in table 2.4 are those set forth by the American College of Sports Medicine (2011) for stretching when it is used as part a fitness programme for healthy adults.

Guidelines for an Active Stretching Programme

- Screen for contraindications.

- Limit the number of recommended stretches to one or two to begin with. Clients are more likely to adhere to a plan that is simple and efficient.

- Explain the rationale for the stretches.

- Demonstrate the stretches and check that the client performs them correctly. Make any necessary adjustments.

- Provide an illustration of each stretch. For example, clients often understand what to do at the time of instruction but later forget where they positioned their feet, whether their knees were supposed to be flexed, whether they were supposed to bear weight through a limb.

- Initially, supervise the stretches. Once you are certain your client is performing these correctly, decrease the amount of supervision you provide.

- Encourage your client to hold each stretch for a minimum of 30 seconds.

- Provide advice on safety.

- Actively discourage the no-pain-no gain approach.

- Reassess.

- Modify any stretches if they prove too difficult for a client to perform or do not seem to be effective in changing posture.

- Document what you are trying to achieve, which stretches you have provided, and any feedback provided by your clients when you next see them. For example, how easy or difficult did they find the stretches? How many times did they manage to perform the stretches? For how long did they hold the stretches?

Table 2.4   Stretching Recommendations

Component	Recommendation
Frequency	2 or more days per week is effective in improving joint range of motion.
Intensity	Effective when the stretch is held at a point of tightness or slight discomfort.
Time	Hold stretches for 10 to 30 seconds; for older adults, holding a stretch 30 to 60 seconds may be more beneficial.
Type	Perform series of exercises for each of the major muscle–tendon units.
Volume	60 seconds total stretching time for each flexibility exercise.
Pattern	Repeat each flexibility exercise 2 or 4 times.
Enhancing	Effectiveness is improved when the muscle is warmed up using light to moderate aerobic exercise or with the application of heat such as with heat packs or hot baths.

- A stretching diary can be useful.

- Develop a portfolio of pictures and ideas to help increase the variety of stretches at your disposal. There are many more stretches available than those provided here. For further information, see *Therapeutic Stretching* (Johnson 2014).

Passive stretching can take many forms. Tying together the ankles of a client who has bilateral genu valgum and leaving them this way for 10 minutes was advocated by Tidy in 1944 as a means of gently stretching the soft tissue structures of the lateral sides of the knee. Although likely to be useful, such techniques today raise ethical and safety issues. This example, however, demonstrates the novel approaches to stretching that have been used in correcting postural problems. Traditional passive stretches are applied to a limb or the spine and stretch more than one muscle. Tractioning is a less-used form of passive stretching involving a gentle, sustained pull on a joint, stretching the capsule, ligaments and associated muscles and their tendons. Tractioning may reduce muscle spasm and may reduce adhesions. As with gross passive stretching, tractioning stretches more than one muscle and affects multiple soft tissues. Dry stretching may be a technique more frequently used by manual therapists when working on a small, specific area. The therapist uses the fingers or thumbs to take up the slack in the skin. Holding the skin at the barrier point encourages soft tissues to lengthen. Soft tissue release (STR) is a pin-and-stretch technique in which soft tissues are gently locked; whilst the lock is maintained, the body part is stretched. Muscle energy technique (MET) involves the active contraction of a muscle by the client against a resistive force provided by the therapist before the stretch is performed. These are just some examples of forms of stretching that could be used to lengthen shortened tissues.

Guidelines for a Passive Stretching Programme

- Screen for contraindications. In addition to general contraindications, note that tractioning should not be used with hypermobile clients or those with a history of subluxation or dislocation in the part to be tractioned. Tractioning should not be used where the broad handhold needed for performing the stretch is likely to damage skin.

- Begin with your client positioned comfortably. Explain what you are going to do.

- Encourage your client to breathe normally rather than to hold the breath in anticipation of being stretched.

- Encourage your client to let you know if he has discomfort or pain, and work only within tolerable levels.

- When stretching the limbs, be sensitive as to where you position your hands.

- Take your time. Both the client and body tissues need the opportunity to relax. Experienced therapists can sense when this occurs. Hold stretches for a minimum of 30 seconds. Only after this should you attempt to take the stretch past the barrier point.

- When treating clients for the first time, work cautiously and do less rather than more. Sometimes changes are immediate, but sometimes they occur over time. Even minor alterations to joint position can have dramatic effects physically and emotionally in some clients. In some cases a client may have soreness in muscles; you should advise the client on this and reassure him that this usually resolves within about 24 hours.

- Restoration of mobility in muscles exhibiting moderate tightness takes several weeks (Kendall et al. 1993).

SOFT TISSUE RELEASE   This form of stretching involves first shortening and then lengthening the muscle to be stretched whilst a lock is applied to the muscle beginning as close to the origin as possible and working towards the insertion with subsequent stretches. Placing a lock on the soft tissues limits the amount by which they can move and seems to localize the stretch to some parts of the muscle more than others. In many cases this is useful because it enables you to focus attention on specific areas of tightness or adhesions. For more information, see *Soft Tissue Release* (Johnson 2009). The technique is simple:

1. Shorten the muscle that is to be stretched. This may be done actively or passively.

2. Choose a point close to the muscle's origin and fix the tissues you intend to stretch using your thumb, fist, forearm or elbow. Avoid pressing into joints or deeply into regions where there are lymph nodes and vascular structures.

3. Whilst maintaining the lock, actively or passively stretch the muscle.

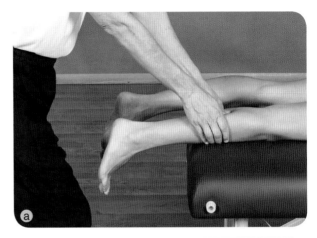

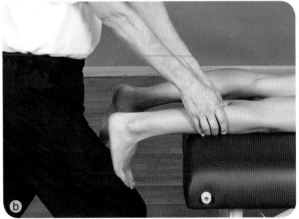

Figure 2.1   Soft tissue release to the calf: *(a)* Apply a gentle lock to the muscle, which already rests in a slightly shortened position when the patient lies prone with feet off the end of the couch; *(b)* maintain the lock as you gently dorsiflex the ankle using your thigh.

MUSCLE ENERGY TECHNIQUE   Muscle energy technique is popularly termed MET. It may be particularly helpful in lengthening postural muscles prone to shortening. It involves the active contraction of a muscle by the client against a resistive force provided by the therapist. The active contraction provided by the client could be beneficial in strengthening muscles and decreases tone in the opposing muscle group. It is not clear what degree of force the client should use, but this should be no more than 25% of the client's maximal force capacity. There are many variations on this technique. One suggested protocol is described here:

1. Position the client so that both you and he are comfortable. Take the muscle to be stretched to a resistance barrier, that point where both you and the client feel an increase in the client's tissues to further elongation. This barrier is the point at which you will start to stretch. Tell your client to let you know as soon as you reach the barrier, a point where he may feel a very slight stretch. The entire procedure should be pain free.

2. Ask the client to contract his muscle (i.e., the one in which he feels the slight stretch) using a maximum of 25% of his muscular force whilst you resist this contraction. Maintain the body part that is being stretched in a static position so the effect is an isometric contraction of the muscle you are about to stretch. It is important that the client be the one who sets the level of contraction against which you resist, not the converse. That is, clients should never resist your force; you should resist theirs.

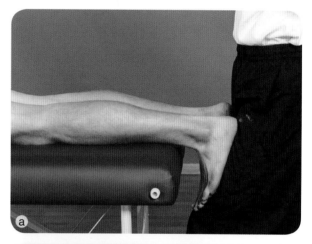

3. After about 10 seconds, ask the client to relax; within the next 3 to 5 seconds, gently ease the body part further into the stretch so you find a new barrier position. Maintain this position for a few seconds before repeating the procedure up to two more times.

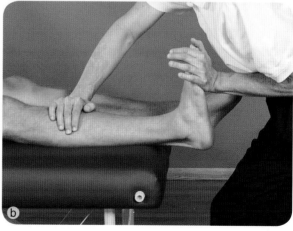

Figure 2.2   Muscle energy technique to the calf: (a) MET to the calf with the client prone, and (b) MET to the calf with the client supine.

Massage

If the degree of muscle tone is a factor determining the lengthening of muscle, then a reduction in tone may result in a greater ability to lengthen a muscle, whether by stretch or by massage. Massage reduces muscle tone and increases general flexibility. Deep tissue massage may improve joint range and the stretching and compressive components used as part of trigger point deactivation. The decrease in muscle tone resulting from some types of massage could be helpful before stretching, and stripping-type techniques may help with the adherence of scar tissue. Tapotement techniques could also stimulate muscles before strengthening exercises. No matter what style of massage is used, when applied for the purposes of postural correction, it could be considered *therapeutic* massage—the 'manipulation of soft tissues of the body by a trained therapist as a component of a holistic therapeutic intervention' (Holey and Cook 2003, p. 6).

It is not known how firmly, for how long in a single bout or how frequently massage should be used to facilitate a lengthening of soft tissues for the purposes of postural correction, as is apparent when you look at table 2.5. Some studies reveal an improvement in joint range due to an increase in muscle length after massage, but massage protocols have varied, making comparisons difficult and the formulation of a massage-for-muscle-lengthening protocol challenging. For more information on the use of deep tissue massage, see *Deep Tissue Massage* (Johnson 2010).

Table 2.5   Suggestions for Frequency and Timing of Massage to Lengthen Muscles

Component	Recommendation
Depth	It is unknown whether massage designed to lengthen muscles is more effective when it is applied using light pressure or deep pressure.
Technique	It is unknown which techniques—effleurage or petrisage, for example—are most effective in lengthening muscles. Not all muscles can be massaged as easily using the same technique, and variations in type of technique used are inevitable.
Duration	It is unknown for how long massage needs to be applied to a particular muscle in order to be effective at lengthening it.
Frequency	It is unknown how frequently massage as a treatment is required to help lengthen a muscle.
Progression	It is unknown how many treatment sessions are required for the use of massage to help lengthen a muscle. This is likely to depend on the existing state of muscle tone and the degree to which it is required to be lengthened, as well as whether there is any underlying pathology, and whether massage is combined with other techniques (e.g., stretching or trigger point deactivation).

Guidelines for Using Massage to Lengthen Shortened Tissues

- Screen your client for contraindications.

- Identify the tissues to be lengthened. Take baseline measurements before the treatment.

- Explain your proposed treatment to the client.

- If necessary, use heat before treatment to increase extensibility of tissues.

- Start with general, slow strokes as you would with any massage and gradually build up to deeper and deeper strokes.

- Encourage feedback from your client. Encourage your client to let you know if she has discomfort or pain, and work only within tolerable levels.

- Resist overworking one area because this can induce soreness. Where possible, link the entire limb, massaging parts above and below. For example, when attempting to lengthen hamstrings, massage the calf distally and the buttocks and back superiorly; when massaging the hip flexors, massage the quadriceps and tibialis anterior distally as well as the abdomen superiorly.

- When treating clients for the first time, work cautiously and do less rather than more.

- Retest the length of the muscle after treatment.

- Document any of the client's adverse reactions (e.g., bruising) in your next session.

Deactivation of Trigger Points

Trigger points are palpable areas of tension that refer pain to other regions and represent localized areas of hypersensitivity within a muscle. They are considered representative of dysfunction in the muscle; they are also associated with postural deficiencies (Huguenin 2004). Muscles found to contain trigger points may exhibit tightness that limits lengthening of the muscle. Therefore, deactivation of the trigger point is believed to help restore more normal muscle functioning and may help address hypomobility in joints associated with that muscle. Many techniques have been described as being useful in the treatment of trigger points, including dry needling, injection with an anaesthetic block, ice cube massage, stretching after cooling with coolant spray, deep massage, myofascial manipulation, reflex inhibition after isometric contraction and laser therapy. For effective treatment of trigger points it seems likely that a multifaceted approach is needed (Hertling and Kessler 2006). The technique described here is for deep tissue massage because it has been found to be one of the most effective forms of treatment for trigger points (Chaitow 2001), and it falls within the remit of massage therapists.

It is not known how many times a trigger point should be pressed using trigger point pressure release in order to deactivate it, nor how frequent the treatment sessions should be (see table 2.6). Nor is it known what degree of pressure should be applied, because pain thresholds vary among individuals. It is likely, however, that excessive pressure will be counterproductive, because trigger points are more susceptible to mechanical trauma than trigger-free muscle is, and if pain occurs, this may cause muscle spasm and the patient to remain tense.

Table 2.6   Suggestions for Frequency and Timings of Trigger Point Pressure Release

Component	Recommendation
Repetitions	It is unknown how many times a trigger point needs to be pressed in order to release it. In some cases the muscle may respond immediately; in others the technique may be ineffective, and repeated attempts at the application of pressure will not bring about a reduction in symptoms.
Intensity	Pressure may be uncomfortable but should not cause pain.
Time	It is unknown how long a treatment session needs to be in order to be effective. In practice, it is likely that this is restricted by the usual time allocated to treatment sessions, such as 1 hour. However, it may be neither necessary nor desirable to attempt to use trigger point pressure release for that length of time on one muscle. In some cases the muscle may respond immediately and treatment is complete; in others the technique may be ineffective and so no length of time will bring about a reduction in symptoms.
Progression	Unknown. It may be that 10 treatment sessions are required in order to relieve the signs and symptoms associated with trigger points. However, this will vary depending on the chronicity of the muscle and how it responds to treatment. Other factors may hinder resolution of symptoms and lengthening of muscle: if the client is self-treating and fails to stretch the muscle tissues after treatment; if the client engages in a physical activity that perpetuates the trigger point; because the formation of trigger points is unclear, food substances or medications could be contributing factors as might other things that affect muscle physiology (e.g., emotional stress, hormones, hydration).

Technique for Treating Trigger Points Using Pressure Point Release

1. Position your client so that the muscle to be treated is lengthened and relaxed.

2. Using palpation, identify the palpable band of tissue in which the trigger point to be treated is located. These are methods of palpation described by Lavelle and colleagues (2007):

   - Flat palpation involves pushing the skin over the affected muscle to one side and sliding the fingertip across the muscle first in one direction and then in the opposite direction. Snapping palpation, as if plucking a string instrument, is then used to identify a specific trigger point.

   - Pincher palpation involves pinching a roll of skin between the finger and thumb and rolling it in order to locate the taut band.

   - Deep palpation is used to identify trigger points that are less superficial. Pressure is applied to one fixed spot at a time until replication of the client's symptoms is elicited; this indicates the presence of the trigger point.

3. Apply pressure to the trigger point gently. Gradually increase pressure until there is a palpable release of tension. Pressure usually elicits mild discomfort but should not be unduly painful. It is thought that the reduction in palpable tension corre-

sponds with equalization of sarcomere length in the muscle and that this can be checked by noting whether there is an increased range of motion (Simons 2002).

4. Repeat this process on the next band of taut tissue.

5. After treatment, stretch the muscle you have been working on.

The technique may be modified to trigger point massage technique. This could involve gentle, short strokes over the point using alternate thumb pressure. Alternatively, the technique could be combined with the lock-and-stretch method used by soft tissue release described in the section on stretching. Instead of selecting a random point to lock tissues, you could select a trigger point and apply gentle stretch whilst maintaining pressure on the spot in question, thus combining both techniques. The client could also take an active role in deactivating trigger points. A home programme consisting of isch-aemic compression of trigger points (as described previously) and sustained stretching has been found to be effective in reducing trigger points (Hanten et al. 2000). Advise your client on using a tennis ball, for example, to press gently into trigger points, avoid-ing pressing into joints themselves, directly onto bone or for too long. Remember that trigger points are a symptom. The increased tension with which they are correlated is likely to persist if the causal factors are not addressed. The key to successful treatment is addressing precipitating and predisposing factors for your client (Huguenin 2004).

Muscle Strengthening

The kinds of muscle strengthening used in postural correction are highly specific as opposed to the overall strengthening you might envision when someone attends a gym to use free weights or multigym equipment. When correcting posture, it is necessary for the client to focus on a specific muscle and to practice contraction of the muscle.

Massage techniques known as tapotement techniques promote an increase in muscle tone. In the initial stages tapotement may be useful in strengthening muscles by helping a client to focus attention on the muscle that needs activation. Tapotement involves short, sudden striking of the skin, which can be very gentle or can be brisk, as in the case of hacking, clapping and beating techniques. These kinds of strokes are stimulating in nature, aimed at increasing vasodilation, vibrating tissues and stimulat-ing cutaneous reflexes.

There are no agreed-on protocols on the use of muscle strengthening for the specific aim of correcting posture. The American College of Sports Medicine (2011) has some evidence-based recommendations (see table 2.7) for resistance exercise when it is used as part a fitness programme for healthy adults; these guidelines can be used as a starting point. When muscle strength training is used to correct posture, the type of training most likely to be effective is endurance training (i.e., training muscles to perform the same movement over a prolonged period). For general fitness, resistance exercises involving each major muscle group are recommended. However, for postural training it is important to be highly selective in which muscles are trained—increasing the endur-ance of shortened or hypertonic muscles will be counterproductive. Similarly, we do not know how best to progress muscle endurance exercise when it is used specifically to aid postural correction. Increasing the number of repetitions per set or increasing the frequency may be beneficial. Regular postural assessment is necessary in order to monitor change and adjust which muscles should be trained.

Table 2.7   Evidence-Based Recommendations on Resistance Exercise

Component	Recommendation
Frequency	Muscle should be trained 2 or 3 days per week.
Intensity	Less than 50% of the 1-repetition max (light to moderate intensity) to improve muscular endurance.
Time	Most effective duration of training is unknown.
Type	For general fitness, use resistance exercises involving each major muscle group.
Repetitions	15 to 20 repetitions improve endurance.
Sets	2 or fewer sets improve muscular endurance.
Pattern	Rest 2 to 3 minutes between each set of repetitions. Rest 48 hours or more between sessions for a single muscle group.
Progression	For general fitness, progress gradually with greater resistance, or more repetitions per set, or increased frequency.

One of the problems with trying to correct posture is that muscles that have become lengthened and weak may remain weak, providing less stability around a joint. Therefore, strengthening exercises—which may involve weight bearing or loading of a joint—need to be performed cautiously. Stretch weakness results from muscles remaining in an elongated position beyond the neutral rest position but within the normal range of muscle length. Muscles often affected by stretch weakness are gluteus medius, gluteus minimus, iliopsoas, hip external rotators, abdominal muscles and lower trapezius (Kendall et al. 1993). Where lengthening of muscle is the result of eccentric contraction, it cannot be reduced by fibre remodelling or exercise training due to structural damage to fibres, possibly the result of shearing in myosin cross bridges (Panel on Musculoskeletal Disorders and the Workplace Commission on Behavioral and Social Sciences and Education National Research Council and Institute of Medicine 2011).

Guidelines for Teaching Clients Muscle Strengthening

- Address any tightness in the opposing muscle first.
- Help your client identify the muscle to be strengthened by touching it.
- Use brisk tapotement techniques, avoiding bone, to stimulate the muscle.
- Ask your client to contract the muscle by giving instructions in layperson terms. For example, rather than instructing to retract rhomboids, ask your client to gently draw their shoulder blades together. Palpate the muscle as your client contracts it, making sure she is performing the exercise correctly.
- The aim of strengthening is to shorten lengthened muscles so that they hold a joint in a more optimal position permanently. Therefore, the ultimate aim is for your client to build up endurance in the exercise until the new posture becomes habitual. One way is to encourage your client to practice holding the contraction for longer and longer periods. In many cases a client will quickly fatigue. Discour-

age the use of maximal contractions. Instead, suggest practicing little and often.

- Advise your client that, as with most forms of strengthening, it is possible they may will have some muscle soreness initially, which usually resolves itself within 24 hours.

- Where necessary, use taping or bracing to maintain alignment until a weak muscle recovers strength. Muscles affected by stretch weakness should be immobilized in the physiological rest position long enough for recovery to occur (Kendall et al. 1993).

- Advise your client that to retain the gain in strength she needs to avoid overworking that particular muscle or falling back into bad postural or occupational habits.

- Participation in a total-body physical activity such as swimming is beneficial for many clients with sedentary occupations. Encourage this unless it aggravates the posture you are trying to correct. For example, discourage clients with increased cervical lordosis (see chapter 3) from holding the head up whilst swimming breaststroke; rowing could aggravate a kyphotic posture (see chapter 4) and is less suitable to clients with shortened hip flexors (read the information on increased lumbar lordosis in chapter 5 and anterior pelvic tilt in chapter 7).

Taping

Taping can correct posture by relieving stress on overstretched tissues and by guiding soft tissues into a new position, or the tension can be used as a behaviour reminder (Hertling and Kessler 2006). There is a danger of clients becoming reliant on the application of tape, believing it to be essential for correcting posture. Self-correction of joints is preferable to taping because self-correction strengthens weakened muscles that are needed for keeping joints in alignment, whereas taping is useful, but only in the short term. The two types of tape are rigid and elastic. Elastic tape is advocated for use in postural correction because it does not limit movement entirely and is more comfortable than rigid tape. The use of elastic tape is a newer practice than the use of rigid tape, and evidence for application for use in postural correction is lacking. Elastic tape, however, is popular among many clinicians who report beneficial results for their clients. There are various texts available for further information, such as that by Langendoen and Sertel (2011). The guidelines provided here are general. Always follow manufacturers' recommendations for the kind of elastic tape you are using.

Guidelines for Taping

- Realign the joint to be taped into a neutral position either passively or actively.
- Ensure the area is free from hair, oil and sweat.
- Stretch the tape slightly before application. The tape will retract on application, pulling the skin with it and helping to keep a joint in the neutral position.
- Elastic tape can be worn for up to a week and should be used for a minimum of three days. Advise the client to remove tape when it is wet, perhaps when showering, gently easing the tape off in the direction of hair growth.

Myofascial Release

Tension in fascia restricts movement and may aggravate abnormal postures. When fascia is consistently overloaded it binds down, creating further postural imbalance, and restricts not only physical structures but thoughts, memory and reactions that may have occurred at the time of injury (Duncan 2014). Myofascial release is a distinct therapy that acts on fascia and may be significant in helping to correct posture by facilitating a more

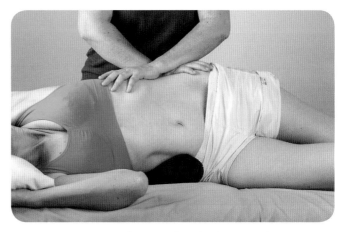

Figure 2.3   Position for cross-hand release to the lateral low back area.

optimal resting position for tissues. During this technique there is a kind of relaxing of tissues—a release in the holding pattern of fascia—and as a result muscles may be better realigned. There are many types of massage and strokes as well as forms of myofascial release. A very basic cross-hand technique is described here. For more detailed information, including a greater variety of techniques in this discipline, see *Myofascial Release* by Ruth Duncan (2014), on which these guidelines are based.

Guidelines for Myofascial Cross-Hand Release Technique

- With crossed hands, gently place your palms on the client's skin and apply gentle, sustained pressure.
- Feel for the resistance beneath your palms until the simple weight of your hands results in a yielding of fascia.
- Wait again at this point, sensing the tissue barrier, and in time your hands should sink slightly further into it.
- As you gently lean onto the client, maintain palm pressure and move your hands apart, taking up the slack in soft tissues.

This technique takes a minimum of 5 minutes, and the release of fascia may occur in one, two or three planes.

Aftercare

When treating a client for postural correction, it is likely that the time between your treatment sessions will become greater. When treatment has reached a stage where the malalignment has been corrected or where no further change in posture seems likely, you need to be certain that the client does not fall back into bad habits. It is worth reiterating the points in the previously mentioned list Helping Your Client Identify,

Eliminate or Reduce Causal Habits and perhaps offering your client a check-up in 6 months. You may have already helped the client to identify primary contributing factors; often a client's new body awareness may make him question whether a particular type of office seating, sport or recreational activity will adversely affect posture. By the time that you discharge the client, the hope is that she will no longer require your input in managing posture. Education regarding the client's condition is paramount from the onset. In some cases there may be nothing further you can do—your client may have a progressively arthritic ankle, for example, and awaiting ankle replacement surgery. You may have taught the client about stretches for muscles in the lower limb and how to overcome compensatory calf cramping, but can offer no further treatment or advice regarding ankle posture.

In subsequent chapters you will note that treatment ideas are listed according to what the therapist can do and what the client can do. The client can participate in postural correction in the following ways:

- Identifying factors contributing to posture
- Modifying behaviour to remove or reduce these factors where possible
- Following your advice for active stretching of specific muscles
- Following your advice for strengthening specific muscles
- Using a tennis ball or other device for deactivating trigger points with the aim of lengthening muscles
- Following other advice that you have discussed with the client (e.g., adopting specific resting posture, avoiding certain types of footwear, changing the method of carrying a backpack, working with another professional such as a sport therapist or podiatrist)

Many of the suggestions for what the client can do could be carried on once face-to-face appointments with you have finished. Indeed, it is likely that many clients will need to continue with a regular programme of stretching or deactivation of trigger points or strengthening in order to counter the effects of a sport or regular physical activity that might be perpetuating a particular posture.

Gaining Rapport and Enhancing Engagement

Ensuring that your client carries out the home care programme you devise is important in bringing about postural change. For example, where compliance to exercise prescribed by a chiropractor is high, results tend to be positive, and therapeutic goals are attained. When compliance is low, therapeutic outcomes may plateau or reverse (Milroy and O'Neil 2000). Unfortunately, compliance to physical therapy is poor, and the reasons for this are extensive and varied. The reasons for non-compliance to supervised exercise found by Sluijs, Kok and van der Zee (1993) were barriers perceived by patients (such as lack of time), lack of positive feedback and feelings of helplessness (where the client believes he can do little to help oneself). These authors recommend that we not assume that we know the reason for non-compliance, nor should we overlook the problems people face when trying to make changes in habits. Whether the findings of Sluijs and colleagues can be attributed to clients prescribed exercise as part of treatment for postural correction is unknown. Postural correction clients may be more strongly motivated to adhere to their programmes. Or, like the majority of patients, they may lack motivation in participation in a home exercise programme. Getting and retaining rapport are paramount. When carrying out an initial postural assessment, noticing the features that do *not* need to be changed (i.e., pointing out the positive features of your client) is likely to help build rapport (Earls and Myers 2010). Also, it is useful to encourage your client to make notes about achievements rather than failures because this is likely to enhance the treatment programme. For example, in addition to admitting to having missed some days of stretching or strengthening, what could your client report she *did* achieve? Did she change her office chair? Did she remember to avoid locking out the knees into hyperextension whilst waiting for the train? Did she manage to sleep on her back instead of their front for part of the week?

You can increase the likelihood of engagement by setting patient-centred goals. Patient-centred care advocates that an understanding of the patient's perspective should underpin good practice in an equal therapeutic relationship (Kidd et al. 2011). People are more likely to have positive treatment outcomes if goals are meaningful to them and they can believe attainment will make a positive change in their lives. Randall and McEwen (2000) recommend the following steps to goal setting:

1. Determine the patient's desired outcome of therapy.
2. Develop an understanding of the patient's self-care, work and leisure activities.
3. Establish goals with the patient that relate to the desired outcomes.

Health care professionals can improve the likelihood that a client will maintain an exercise behaviour by giving supportive feedback and instructing clients on self-monitoring and goal setting (Woodard and Berry 2001). It is likely that many more methods over and above face-to-face advice and treatment are needed for fully engaging clients. Information technology provides an ever-growing and diverse means of communicating information to clients and may help some adhere to treatment programmes. In *Personal Health Information Technology—Paradigm for Providers and Patients to Transform Healthcare Through Patient Engagement*, Sarasohn-Kahn (2013) gives a variety of examples of personal health information technology, including Skyping, mobile apps, e-mail, and social networks for patient peer-to-peer support. With increasing reliance on clients' taking responsibility for their own rehabilitation, you could consider how you might adapt information technology for use with the correction of posture. How could you increase the likelihood of your clients' fully engaging with the postural correction programme you and he devise?

Referral to Another Practitioner

At times all therapists need to refer clients to other health care practitioners, either because the therapist considers that treatment of factors causing or contributing to the posture in question falls outside his or her professional remit or because the client is not responding to treatment as might be expected. In some cases it may be more appropriate for a client to receive treatment of a different kind first in order to achieve a more successful outcome. For example, if an obese client with a genu valgum knee posture had a lot of knee pain, and during the consultation reported wanting to reduce weight but is struggling to do so, she may benefit more from advice and support of a dietician than from massage to tensioned tissues around the knee joint. By contrast, a very underweight client with a hyperextending knee, also with knee pain, who reports finding it difficult to eat healthfully might also benefit from input from a dietician; but in this case, taping the posterior knee could provide immediate, albeit temporary, relief from pain that would make it easier for the client to walk before the dietician's appointment. In these examples, the focus is not solely on the body mass index of the patient, and the intention is not to imply that an obese person should be treated by a dietician before hands-on therapy, whereas an underweight person need not receive advice from a dietician. Rather, an obese patient with this specific type of knee posture may benefit more from engaging in weight loss first, because soft tissue treatment or taping is likely to provide only extremely short-term relief; the weight of the body will force the knee into genu valgum posture again on weight bearing. If an obese patient had a hyperextending knee, then it is possible that taping, as a form of temporary postural correction, could be effective because it is easier to conscientiously avoid knee extension in weight bearing and walking than it is to avoid genu valgum. There are no hard-and-fast rules about when to refer, and each case should be decided independently. The only exception to this is if you suspect your client has a serious pathology such as undiagnosed cancer, in which case you should refer the client immediately to a medial doctor.

Table 2.8 contains a list of some health care providers along with examples of when referral may be indicated. The list of providers is not exhaustive; many more examples could be included for each as reasons for referral. To whom you choose to refer may depend on whom you know, or you may be working in a practice where there are clear referral pathways set out, with guidelines regarding referral to specific practitioners. If you work as an independent therapist, it is useful to establish a network of like-minded professionals to whom you could refer your clients.

Networking with other therapists in the same line of work as yours can be useful too, because those therapists are likely to have contacts they are willing to share with you. Even where you have a variety of contacts to whom you may refer, it can be difficult to know to whom your client is best suited. For example, the distinction between the skills used by a podiatrist and a dentist is clear, whereas the distinction between the skills of two soft tissue therapists may not be: Hands-on therapists usually begin training in Swedish massage but often extend their repertoire to become competent in more than one type of hands-on therapy. Additionally, there is much overlap in the skills used by some health care providers. For example, sport massage may be provided by a sports massage therapist or by a sport therapist, and some physiotherapists, osteopaths and chiropractors are likely to be trained in this skill too. A massage therapist skilled in myofascial release techniques does not have the skill set of a physiotherapist, yet some physiotherapists are trained in myofascial release techniques and may be using this

Table 2.8   Health Care Professionals and Reasons for Referral

Professional	Reasons for referral
Chiropodist, podiatrist	When you observe that the toes or toenails of your client may be adversely affecting foot posture; where your client has an underlying pathology such as arthritis or diabetes affecting the feet; where the use or orthotics may be indicated; where calluses, corns or painful verrucas affect weight bearing.
Physio-therapist, chiropractor, osteopath	These professionals diagnose, treat and manage conditions that are due to problems with muscles, joints, ligaments, tendons and nerves. Whether you refer to a chiropractor, osteopath or physiotherapist may depend on personal preference or, in some cases and countries, may be determined by matters of insurance (where therapeutic treatment is paid for by an insurance agency). Physiotherapists in particular have advanced knowledge of rehabilitation and may specialize in a particular field (e.g., women's health, elderly care, neurology), so referral could be based on whether your client falls into one of these categories. Referral may be appropriate where your client has an underlying and poorly controlled condition that is likely to affect postural correction (e.g., a neurological condition such as multiple sclerosis). Or where the postural deformity results from injury or surgical intervention and rehabilitation is required; where mobilization or manipulation of joints is likely to be beneficial as part of the treatment; where mobilization of neural tissue is warranted.
Counsellor	Where the posture in question causes your client embarrassment or where there are other concerns about body image; where an emotional issue is hindering postural correction.
Dentist	Where a client with a forward head posture reports temporomandibular joint pain.
Doctor	Where pain limits postural correction, a doctor is best placed to advise on pain management; when referral to an additional specialist is needed—in the UK it is usual for a patient to be referred to a doctor who then assesses whether referral to a specialist (such as a physiotherapist or podiatrist) is the most favourable course of action; when you suspect a serious pathology.
Fitness instructor, personal trainer	Where you and your client decide that he would benefit from receiving one-to-one supervision when carrying out tailored muscle strengthening or stretching programme; where you and your client agree that participation in a weight loss programme will contribute to postural correction.
Massage therapist	Where you discern that hypertonicity in muscles is due in part to stress and deem non-specific, general relaxation massage to be beneficial; where myofascial release may be beneficial.
Sports massage therapist	Where you do not have the additional skills used by many sport massage therapists to decrease muscle tone and lengthen tissues and believe these may be beneficial (e.g., use of muscle energy technique, soft tissue release, trigger point deactivation, deep tissue massage).
Sport therapist	Where the client needs to engage in recreational or professional sporting activity and the posture in question hinders this; where advice on sporting biomechanics is required.

skill with a different client group. If you know that your client is keen to take up sport or is already engaged in regular physical activity, it would be wise to refer the client to a specialist. The American Physical Therapy Association have a special-interest group called the Sports Physical Therapy Section, and members specialize in prevention, evaluation, treatment, rehabilitation and performance enhancement of physically active individuals and carry out postural observations from all angles as part of their examinations (Sanders et al. 2013). In the UK this group is called the Association of Chartered Physiotherapists in Sports and Exercise Medicine. This kind of specialist intervention is also provided in the UK by sport therapists, considered a profession in its own right. Each of these groups can advise on sporting activities likely to aggravate postural imbalance and may even be able to recommend sports that improve posture. There is great benefit in focusing on what you do best and collaborating with practitioners of other disciplines. Governing organizations each provide definitions and descriptions of the professionals they represent; this can help you to determine which professional may be of most help. For example, the Society of Sports Therapists (2013) compares the role of a sports therapist with the role of a physiotherapist, and the Chartered Society of Physiotherapists and Fitness Industry Association Joint Working Party (2011) provides guidelines on choosing between referral to a physiotherapist and referral to a fitness instructor. None of the organizations gives recommendations for referral specifically related to the correction of posture. Bear in mind also that referral need not be to a practitioner of a discipline different to yours. In some cases it may be useful to discuss the client's case with a colleague. Whenever and to whomever you refer, you will require signed consent from your client.

Tailoring Your Treatments

The postures described in this book are varied, and some are more correctable than others. Factors that influence whether a posture is correctable include the underlying cause of the posture, ongoing contributing factors and your client's willingness to engage in the correction process (i.e., willingness to follow advice and to perform the exercise, stretches or treatments that you recommend). Where the desire for change is driven by the client, the outcomes are likely to be more favourable. Intrinsic as opposed to extrinsic motivation is likely to be more long lasting. The frequency with which you provide treatment ultimately depends on the intrinsic motivation of your client to engage in postural change and his or her cognitive ability to do so.

Described as follows are five clients with the same posture—an overly developed kyphotic curve—used to illustrate how you might modify and tailor your treatment to suit each client. There are many examples that could illustrate variations in treatment approaches. In contrast to these examples, the desire for postural change is often derived from the therapist who, as the protagonist, has assessed that a change in posture will reduce existing symptoms or reduce the likelihood of symptoms' developing. In all cases, the desire for the correction—as far as is possible—must be a goal your client agrees. For the actual techniques that you may use to correct a kyphotic posture, see chapter 4.

CASE STUDIES INVOLVING KYPHOTIC CURVE

Client 1 is 6 feet 3 inches (190.5 cm) tall, physically fit and regularly participating in rowing (a hobby he has kept up since university). He reports tending to stoop when speaking to people. He has had some ache in the upper back and was intending to come for a massage anyway. Despite being very busy at work, he has been prompted to make the appointment because, when looking through some recent photos of an office party, he was shocked at how hunched he appeared compared to how he looked in photos of himself a few years ago. He is very keen to know if his posture can be changed or if it is too late. Accustomed to exercise, he is happy to embrace any stretching or strengthening programme you provide. He is looking forward to seeing you for as many sessions as it takes to receive treatment or advice and check on progress.

After the initial appointment, this client reports being keen to avoid the stooped posture and, following your suggestion, agrees to ask his colleagues to remind him when he slips into his stooping habit. He agrees that meeting with a sport therapist to discuss rowing technique might be helpful and may shed further light on what he can do to correct his kyphotic posture. When you see the client for his second and third appointments, he asks questions and wants to be certain he is performing the stretches correctly. He is able to demonstrate these and reports having practiced them regularly. He is happy to receive hands-on treatment. He has looked up the muscles you described at the first appointment and understands your treatment rationale. Overall, he is actively engaged in the process of his postural correction.

Client 2 is physically unfit and has noticed her posture has deteriorated since starting her new job a few years ago in a call centre. She admits to struggling with self-confidence and reports feeling that this is one of the reasons her posture is poor, because she tends to hunch over a little when speaking with people with whom she feels self-conscious. You discuss treatment options; she reports feeling very uncomfortable with the idea of receiving hands-on treatment but is willing to do some stretches.

When you see this client for her second appointment, she has not performed the stretches you prescribed and admits to not having changed her posture much at all during the day. She reports feeling too embarrassed to stand up straight when speaking with people in the office and feeling too tired to stretch when she gets home. During some exploratory questioning, you discover that this client is willing to commit to making behavioural changes but feels she needs more guidance on it. You provide her with a 7-day diary sheet with pictures of the muscles to be stretched and boxes for her to check when she has completed the stretch. She likes this and feels that by keeping the diary in the kitchen she will see it daily and use it to help monitor her progress. You agree to see her weekly, a schedule she prefers. You return to the question of her self-consciousness and ask with whom she *would* feel confident standing up tall in order to have a conversation: a family member? A friend? The ticket collector at the bus depot? The person who delivers the mail? She agrees to identifying the number of opportunities each day she gets to engage in conversation with someone with whom she feels comfortable standing up straight to speak with and documenting this.

When your client returns the following week, she reports having consciously improved her standing posture three or four times since your previous session and having made the effort when feeling less self-conscious. You discuss what she would need to do to continue with this on a more frequent basis. She has performed the stretches on five occasions and brings her diary in which she has documented this. She has a couple questions about the stretches.

In subsequent weeks this client becomes more confident with stretching and reports improving her posture at least once daily. She would still prefer not to receive any hands-on treatment, so you agree that her postural change programme will involve self-management using stretches and later some strengthening exercises. At this time she does not feel confident enough to attend a gym or to see a personal trainer. She does, however, like your suggestion to ask her manager about having her work station assessed and understands that the height of her computer screen and her manner of sitting all day at work could be hindering the correction of her kyphotic posture.

When you see her the following week, your client has received an assessment by the company's DSE (display screen equipment) assessor and adjustments have been implemented. Apparently her chair was positioned too high and her screen too low, and she was hunching over as she typed in an attempt to see the screen.

Several months later, having practiced these with you on several occasions, she was performing some very simple strengthening exercises at home (again recording these in a diary), which she preferred to attending a public gym. This client lacked confidence and initially required more therapeutic support but was eventually happy to reduce the frequency of her appointments.

Client 3 has Down syndrome and attends the appointment with his carer because during a welfare meeting he expressed an interest in improving the appearance of his back. He has noticed that many of the residents in the care home where he lives are 'round backed' and he thinks he is getting round backed and doesn't like it. He is already participating in a group exercise class at a local health centre once per week, which is run by a specialist exercise instructor, and he enjoys it. The stretching and exercise sheets that you usually give to clients with kyphosis are not suitable for this client because the type size you have selected is rather small and he has some difficulty seeing it. You, your client and the carer all practice a chest stretch, once in standing and once in the supine position. Your client tells you that they do some stretches during his exercise class. Together you decide that one option is to ask the exercise instructor whether she would consider adding some pectoral stretches to the programme as well as some rhomboid retraction exercises, if the instructor thought this was appropriate for the class as a whole.

(continued)

Case Studies Involving Kyphotic Curve *(continued)*

Your client wants to know if there is anything else to help prevent him from being round backed. You explain that chest stretches can be helpful when these are provided by a therapist. With the permission of the client's carer you demonstrate a muscle energy technique stretch on the carer. Your client wishes to receive the stretch but finds difficulty relaxing, and you realize that your instruction was not clear enough because once in the stretch position, the client attempts to stretch *you* rather than receive the stretch himself. The carer asks whether you would consider visiting the home to take part in the monthly wellness session; each month there is a different topic and demonstration and she wonders if you could contribute on the topics of posture, massage and stretching. You agree with your client that this would be a good way to continue his treatment, because you could have his review appointments at the care home rather than have him come to your clinic.

Client 4 works long hours as a stable hand, which involves regular unloading of equipment and much cleaning of stables. She tells you that her friends have noticed she is 'getting a hump' on her back, which she never used to have. She has recently taken up dressage because she thinks it might improve her posture. She requests that you check her posture fully to make sure the hump is nothing serious and to make any necessary recommendations. Your assessments reveal an increase in the kyphotic curve of the upper thorax with shortened abdominal and hip flexor muscles and hypertonic rhomboids on one shoulder. Her shoulder adductor muscles (notably latissimus dorsi) are particularly tight. Your client says she would mostly like advice on correcting these imbalances herself and admits that she is unwilling to commit to regular treatment. The reason is that she works long hours and lives far from your practice. Also, a massage therapist is supposed to be opening a practice in the village where she lives, so it is likely that she will see that therapist rather than travelling to your office. She is, however, happy to come back for a one-off check-up in about 3 months if that were necessary; during that time she will work on all of the stretches and exercises you have provided. You reassure your client and provide the necessary advice regarding correction of a kyphotic posture. Additionally, you mention that she may wish to consider building some hip flexor and shoulder adductor stretches into her programme in the future, and you explain the rationale for this. You recommend that her review appointment be in 6 weeks rather than 12 because it is important to check that she is performing the stretches correctly. She agrees and ends up returning for a further three appointments, each a month apart, during which you reassess her posture and provide both massage and passive stretches. She has noticed a marked improvement in her posture. It is not clear whether this improvement is the result of your hands-on intervention, her active stretching or her regular participation in dressage classes.

Client 5 has Parkinson's disease and attends your appointments with his wife, who is concerned about her husband's deteriorating posture and balance. Your client is willing to practice the stretches you describe, but he is forgetful. He explains that he and his wife used to live abroad and received weekly massages for many years, which he found beneficial and relaxing. He seems amenable to postural correction, but at the initial appointment you cannot be certain whether he is motivated to perform the exercises or whether he would prefer to receive only massage. You explain that there is both a physiotherapist and an osteopath at the practice where you work and that either could provide guidance on specific exercises for maintaining or improving balance. You explain that the change in posture is likely to be associated with Parkinson's disease and that the kyphosis may become more exaggerated with time, but certain exercises and stretches are likely to slow this process. You explain that improving posture will help improve balance and may be beneficial for helping to keep the rib cage elevated and functioning more optimally than in the kyphotic posture.

At a subsequent appointment, your client reports feeling fatigued after his balance training sessions with the physiotherapist. In your own treatment sessions, you have attempted to go through active stretches with your client and to perform some passive stretching. But your client admits to preferring to receive general relaxation massage, so you agree that massage will be the aim of your treatment from now on. You nevertheless focus slightly more on reducing tension in shortened muscles whilst incorporating this into a general massage routine. Your client continues to practice his stretches daily at home under the guidance of his wife.

Table 2.9 illustrates the case of a client with rotation of the neck. This example illustrates how postural correction for one particular part of the body might be treated over the course of five sessions. In this particular example, the client's symptoms may be due to tension in the muscles used to bring about this rotation. How information is recorded varies among therapists. You may be accustomed to using the headings Aggravating Factors or Easing Factors to document subjective symptoms, and the recording of symptoms may be on a body chart or scale. In this example, SOAP notes are used. SOAP notes are one means of recording clinical information:

- Subjective: What your client says about the problem or intervention
- Objective: Your objective observations and treatment tests
- Assessment: Your analysis of the various components of the assessment
- Plan: How the treatment will be developed to reach the goals or objectives

Only summary details are provided. In this example are five sessions spread across 8 weeks.

Table 2.9   SOAP Notes Taken Over a Series of Five Treatments

SOAP notes	Session 1
Subjective	**Problem:** Four-month history of insidious right-sided neck pain since changing desk position at work. Pain described as aching, initially intermittent but now constant, around 5 or 6 on a scale of 10, sometimes burning worsened when at desk for an hour. Time of onset of neck pain at work is gradually decreasing; now has pain after sitting for about 40 minutes. Pain worsens as day progresses; one episode of right arm aching after an 8-hour day at work and resolved on taking hot bath, but now neck pain persists into evening. **Treatment to date:** Doctor diagnosed postural strain and prescribed painkillers and rest. Heat previously helped but no longer helps. Analgesics dull pain but do not resolve it. Otherwise well; no other medical issues. **Patient expectations:** Wants to know if there is anything other than painkillers and rest that can be done to ease neck pain.
Objective	■ Slight rotation of head and neck to right side when viewed both anteriorly and posteriorly, possibly 2 to 5 degrees. ■ Active neck range of motion full but with pulling sensation in right side of neck on rotation to left and on left lateral flexion. ■ Hypertonicity in right scalenes and upper trapezius with trigger points present. ■ Shortening of right levator scapulae. ■ Some tenderness on palpation of left sternocleidomastoid. ■ Shoulder range of motion normal.
Assessment	■ Right-sided neck pain due to muscular imbalance of cervical rotators, possibly aggravated by work posture. ■ **Goals:** Reduce severity and intensity of neck pain from constant 5 or 6 out of 10 to 2 out of 10 intermittent within 7 days using massage initially and programme of daily stretches. ■ Work station assessment to be carried out and adjustments made if necessary. ■ **Treatment:** Treatment rationale explained and treatment agreed on with patient. ■ 5 minutes grade 1 effleurage to upper trapezius and levator scapulae provided, followed by firm petrissage for 5 minutes. Tenderness reported by client. Reduced pulling sensation on re-testing active range of neck motion. Neck pain reduced to 2 or 3 out of 10. Gave advice regarding possible post-massage soreness. ■ Taught client levator scapulae stretch, upper trapezius stretch. Gave illustration of each with guidelines. ■ Explained how to perform deactivation of trigger points using tennis ball.
Plan	■ Client to request work station assessment. ■ Client to perform daily stretches for 1 week per guidelines. ■ Client to practice trigger point release per guidelines. ■ Review appointment in 1 week.

Session 2	
Subjective	No adverse reactions after neck massage in appointment 1. Neck pain reduced to 2 out of 10 the night of the first treatment. However, right-side neck pain returned next day and continues to be around 5 or 6 out of of 10 after sitting for about 40 minutes at desk. Has managed to stretch on occasion during day and has temporary reduction in pain to about 2 out of 10 afterwards for about 10 minutes until pain returns. Pain still worsens as day progresses. Continues to take analgesics as prescribed by doctor. Not yet managed to practice self-triggering of affected muscles. Has requested work station assessment and manager agreed to organize this.
Objective	Findings unchanged: ■ Slight rotation of head and neck to right side when viewed both anteriorly and posteriorly. ■ Active neck range of motion full but with pulling sensation in right side of neck on rotation to left and on left lateral flexion. ■ Hypertonicity in right scalenes and upper trapezius with trigger points present. ■ Shortening of right levator scapulae. ■ Some tenderness on palpation of left sternocleidomastoid.
Assessment	■ Ongoing right-side neck pain due to muscular imbalance of cervical rotators, possibly aggravated by work posture. Patient requires additional support to help build in self-care. ■ **Goals:** Reduce severity and intensity of neck pain from constant 5 or 6 out of 10 to 2 out of 10 intermittent within 7 days. ■ Assess work station and make adjustments if necessary. ■ **Treatment:** Treatment rationale explained and treatment agreed on with patient. ■ 5 minutes grade effleurage to upper trapezius and levator scapulae provided, followed by firm petrissage for 5 minutes. Tenderness reported by client. Three trigger points identified in right levator scapulae and treated. Passive levator scapulae stretch applied in supine; passive upper trapezius stretch in supine. No further pulling sensation on re-testing active range of neck motion. Neck pain 0 out of 10 after treatment. ■ Discussed value of self-deactivation of trigger points. Client agreed to usefulness in pain reduction. ■ Praised client for having attempted stretches. ■ Praised client for having requested work station assessment.
Plan	■ Client to perform stretches for 2 weeks. ■ Client to attempt to self-trigger on 3 occasions each week. ■ Review appointment in 2 weeks.

(continued)

Table 2.9   *(continued)*

Session 3	
Subjective	No adverse reactions after neck massage or stretches in appointment 2. Had 2 out of 10 neck pain that night, much reduced from normal. Right-side neck pain returned next day and continued to be around 5 or 6 out of 10 after sitting for about 40 minutes at desk; has managed to do stretches more regularly, about twice daily, and continues to have only temporary reduction in pain to about 2 out of 10 afterwards, for about 10 minutes until pain returns. Pain still worsens as day progresses. Work station assessment was carried out and assessor recommended moving computer monitor from right side of desk so that it is centralized. Facilities management made this change mid-week. From mid-week, neck pain intermittent. Longer-lasting relief from stretching, up to 30 minutes where pain reduced to 2 out of 10. Practiced self-triggering over weekend and was pain free during this time. Has stopped taking analgesics. On return to work after weekend, neck pain much reduced but had 3 or 4 out of 10 pain by end of day for 3 days.
Objective	Postural findings unchanged: ■ Slight rotation of head and neck to right side when viewed both anteriorly and posteriorly. Other findings: ■ Active neck range of motion full with mild pulling sensation in right side of neck on rotation to left; on left lateral flexion client reports less pulling than normal. ■ Hypertonicity in right scalenes and upper trapezius. ■ Shortening of right levator scapulae. ■ Tenderness on palpation of left sternocleidomastoid reported to be reduced from previous weeks.
Assessment	Right-side neck pain due to muscular imbalance of cervical rotators reducing. Work posture likely contributing factor. Symptoms reducing but no change in posture. ■ **Goals:** Reduce severity and intensity of neck pain from intermittent 3 or 4 of 10 to 0 of 10 intermittent within 7 days. ■ **Treatment:** Treatment rationale explained and treatment agreed on with patient. ■ 5 minutes grade effleurage to upper trapezius and levator scapulae provided, followed by firm petrissage for 5 minutes. Tenderness reported by client. Reduced pulling sensation on re-testing active range of neck motion. Neck pain reduced to 1 out of 10. ■ Observed client perform levator scapulae and upper trapezius stretches. These have been done correctly. Discussed how to build more stretching into day. Patient agreed to attempt a.m., lunchtime and p.m. stretches. ■ Observed patient demonstrate use of tennis ball for deactivation of trigger points in levator scapulae and trapezius. Reiterated importance of this and gave rationale again. ■ Taught how to rest with head rotated to left, using book for support and stretch. ■ Praised client for having had work station assessment. Discussed importance of centralization of computer screen. Patient reports having television positioned to side of room at home. Advised against watching television with head turned to right. Patient agreed to consider change of seating or moving television.

Plan	▪ Client to perform stretches for 1 week.
	▪ Client to attempt to self-trigger on 3 occasions in week.
	▪ Client to reposition self or television at home when watching TV.
	▪ Review appointment in 2 weeks.

Session 4	
Subjective	No adverse reactions after neck massage or stretches in appointment 3. No neck pain at night. Has not had neck pain until last few hours of day—mild, 1 or 2 out of 10. Practicing stretches 3 times per day. Managed to self-trigger 2 times each week for 2 weeks. Enjoys the neck stretch using book and feels this helps. Has changed seating at home so watches TV centralized rather than looking to right.
Objective	Postural findings unchanged:
	▪ Slight rotation of head and neck to right side when viewed both anteriorly and posteriorly.
	Other findings:
	▪ Active and full range of motion in neck and symptom free.
	▪ Previous hypertonicity in right scalenes and upper trapezius feels reduced.
	▪ Levator scapulae length equal bilaterally.
	▪ Palpation of left sternocleidomastoid pain free.
Assessment	▪ Right-side neck pain due to muscular imbalance of cervical rotators much reduced, from constant 5 or 6 out of 10 to intermittent 1 or 2 out of 10. Patient has made lifestyle changes to habits that appear to contribute to reduction in symptoms. Patient happy with ongoing progress. Understands neck rotation may have been causing symptoms. Eager to maintain correct neck alignment.
	▪ **Goals:** Reduce severity and intensity of neck pain from intermittent 1 or 2 out of 10 to 0 within 7 days.
	▪ **Treatment:** Treatment rationale explained and treatment agreed on with patient.
	▪ Soft tissue release performed 3 times to right scalenes after effleurage for 5 minutes; trigger point release to 3 points in right levator scapulae. Passive stretch of levator scapulae.
	▪ Taught how to palpate own scalenes to determine tonicity. Explained rationale. Taught active soft tissue release of scalenes.
	▪ Discussed importance of taking micro-breaks at work, away from display screen equipment.
Plan	▪ Client to continue with levator scapulae, upper trapezius and resting neck stretches as guided, plus continue with trigger point release as guided.
	▪ Client to practice soft tissue release to scalenes.
	▪ Client to build micro-breaks into daily routine.
	▪ Review appointment in 4 weeks.

(continued)

Table 2.9   *(continued)*

Session 5	
Subjective	No adverse reactions after neck massage or stretches in appointment 4. No further neck pain at work. Has got into routine of performing stretches a.m. and p.m. and taking micro-breaks. Continues to use computer screen centralized. Continues to sit facing TV when watching. Continues to perform trigger point release Mon, Wed, Fri but can no longer feel triggers. Has attempted soft tissue release to scalenes but dislikes stretch sensation on anterior neck so has stopped this activity. Because pain free, does not feel need for further treatment.
Objective	■ Cervical posture appears normal. ■ Active cervical range of motion is full and pain free. ■ Tonicity of upper trapezius and levator scapulae reduced. ■ Left and right levator scapulae length equal bilaterally. ■ Sternocleidomastoid pain free.
Assessment	■ Right-side neck pain due to muscle imbalance of cervical rotators now resolved with programme of self-management and 4 treatment sessions over 8 weeks. Patient has made lifestyle changes and is happy to continue in this manner, along with stretches and trigger point release.
Plan	■ Patient symptom free and happy for discharge.

Closing Remarks

In this chapter five steps are proposed for facilitating postural correction. You have learnt why the identification of causal and perpetuating factors is so important for the correction of posture and why client-led correction may have a greater impact than corrective techniques used by a therapist. The rationale for the use of stretching, massage, strengthening, deactivation of trigger points and taping is discussed, and guidelines are provided for each of these techniques. The importance of gaining rapport and improving engagement with and adherence to therapy is covered. You've learnt examples of when referral to another health care practitioner may be useful. Mini-case studies for five clients all presenting with the same back posture demonstrate how unique treatment approaches were needed for each client. An example of treatment notes reveals how treatment might progress over a 5-week period.

Correcting the Spine

In part II you will learn about 10 postures specific to various regions of the spine and will discover how these are interrelated. The postures covered in chapter 3, Cervical Spine, are increased lordosis, lateral neck flexion, forward head posture and rotation of the head and neck. Chapter 4, Thoracic Spine, includes kyphosis, flatback and rotated thorax. Chapter 5, Lumbar Spine, covers both increased lordosis and decreased lordosis. Chapter 6 is devoted to the scoliotic posture; this affects multiple sections of the spine and is more difficult to treat than the other postures.

Cervical Spine

Learning Outcomes

After reading this chapter, you should be able to do the following:

- List four postures common to the cervical region of the spine.
- Describe the anatomical features of each of these postures.
- Recognize these postures on a client.
- Give examples of the anatomical consequences of each posture.
- Name the muscles that are shortened and those that are lengthened in each posture.
- Give examples of appropriate treatments for the correction of each posture.
- Give the rationale for such treatments and, where relevant, state for which clients a particular treatment is contraindicated and why.
- Give examples of the kinds of stretches, exercises and activities that may be suitable to give to clients with specific postures of the cervical spine and state for which clients these self-management tools might be contraindicated.

The four postures described in this chapter are increased cervical lordosis of the neck, laterally flexed neck, forward head posture, and rotated head and neck posture. Other less frequently observed postures (such as a flattening of the cervical lordosis without the associated forward head posture) are not included here. As you observe clients, you will no doubt discover that the four postures presented in this chapter do not occur in isolation; you might discover a client with a combination of both lateral flexion and rotation of the neck, for example.

Viewed posteriorly, the cervical spine is vertical. Viewed from the side, it is convex anteriorly and concave posteriorly, creating a lordotic curve. This normal lordosis improves the cervical spine's resistance to axial compression. Weighing approximately 10 pounds (4.5 kg), the head and forces associated with head movement are transmitted through the bodies of cervical vertebrae, their associated discs and their facet joints. The position of the head greatly influences the position of the spine, and prolonged alterations in normal posture of the cervical spine are likely to affect the neck's load-bearing capabilities. Non-neutral spinal posture is also likely to fatigue muscles of neck and shoulder stabilization. Changes in head and neck posture are also likely to affect the functioning of the thoracic spine and the shoulders. Clear links have been found between thoracolumbar posture in sitting and head and neck posture (Caneiro et al. 2010). The implication is that in order to bring about change, it is likely that adjustments to the thorax and lumbar regions will be needed in addition to those of the head and neck that are described in this chapter.

Increased Lordosis

An increase in the normal lordotic curve of the cervical spine appears as a kind of squashing down of the neck, as if there were a compression of vertebrae one onto another. Sometimes the increased lordosis is evidenced by a crease at the back of the neck when you view your patient posteriorly.

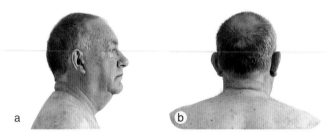

a b

Figure 3.1 (a) An increase in the normal lordotic curve of the cervical spine may appear as a squashing down of the neck when the patient is viewed from the side; (b) in some cases a horizontal crease is present on the back of the neck as in this patient who also demonstrates clockwise rotation of the head.

Table 3.1   Muscle Lengths Associated With Increased Cervical Lordosis

	Shortened muscles	Lengthened muscles
Area	Posterior neck	Anterior neck
Superficial	Upper fibres of trapezius Levator scapulae	Sternocleidomastoid Scalenes
Deep	Semispinalis colli Semispinalis capitis Splenius colli Splenius capitis	Longus capitis Longus colli

Consequences of Increased Lordosis

In this posture the posterior soft tissues of the neck are compressed and the anterior tissues are lengthened. Greater pressure is placed on the posterior aspect of intervertebral discs than on the anterior, and the orientation of facet joints changes. The posterior and anterior longitudinal ligaments are affected: The posterior longitudinal ligament is compressed and the anterior longitudinal ligament is lengthened. The posterior ligament usually helps check neck flexion and covers arteries, veins and lymphatic vessels as they pass into the cancellous bone of the bodies of cervical vertebrae. In flexion, it is normally tensioned, trapping fluid in the cancellous bodies and perhaps facilitating the bone's ability to withstand compression. Could prolonged compression of this ligament that occurs in the lordotic neck posture affect the vascularity of these bones? The anterior longitudinal ligament usually limits neck extension. Together these ligaments exert slight compressional forces on the vertebrae, stabilizing them during movements of the head and neck. Theoretically, lengthening one side of this guy-rope type mechanism, and shortening the other, could adversely affect this function.

It is also postulated that increasing the lordotic curve of the neck results in decreased strength in deep neck flexors. Patients with neck pain are often observed to have poor cervical posture with an increase in the activity of superficial neck flexors and decrease in the activity of deep cervical flexors when performing craniocervical flexion (Falla, Jull, and Hodges 2004).

TIP There is compression of the fascia and skin on the posterior aspect of the neck. The bump, sometimes referred to as a dowager's hump, which can often be seen in the cervicothoracic junction, can indicate tension in tissues of the sternum and a diaphragm that rests low (relative to its optimal resting position). Tension in fascia of the diaphragm and pericardium, attaching to the sternum and up to the neck, could cause a pull on sternocleidomastoid, resulting in this unusual neck posture. Addressing tension in the chest and abdomen could therefore be warranted.

TIP It is also important to examine and address thoracolumbar posture.

What You Can Do as a Therapist

- Begin by encouraging your client to correct posture when sitting or standing by paying particular attention to the spine. To give your client a sense of what it feels like to have a lengthened, more normalized neck posture, you could apply a gentle passive stretch to the neck. Some therapists do this manually by gently placing one hand beneath the chin and one hand on the head as the client rests in the supine position. However, this form of traction can be uncomfortable, and you need to use caution so that you do not overstretch tissues, compress the submandibular glands or extend the head and neck. An alternative is to gently hook one hand beneath the occiput and place the other on the shoulder. Next, apply either gentle traction to the head, or gentle depression of the shoulder, or both (figure 3.2a).

Another alternative is to use a towel, hooking the hemmed edge of the towel beneath the occiput and applying gentle traction (figure 3.2b). This takes practice because sometimes the position of the towel causes the head and neck to extend, and that is counterproductive. With experimentation you will discover which towel placement facilitates the most neutral neck position as you apply traction.

■ Massage shortened tissues, in this case neck extensor muscles. This could be done in supine or prone positions. As you draw your hands from the base of the neck to the head, encourage your client to notice how the lengthening of the neck feels. Resting with your fingertips at the base of the skull, ask your client to make a very small nodding movement because this helps lengthen the short neck extensors (figure 3.2c). Note that this nodding movement is small, different to neck flexion.

In the prone position you can also encourage this gentle nod and stretch of posterior tissues by applying gentle traction to the base of the skull. Asking your client to perform a chin tuck movement helps you gain access to the back of the neck and is especially useful when treating clients with increased adipose tissue in this region.

■ Address trigger points in suboccipital muscles. As you massage and gently stretch posterior tissues, you are likely to identify trigger points. These may be addressed with gentle pressure (figure 3.2d).

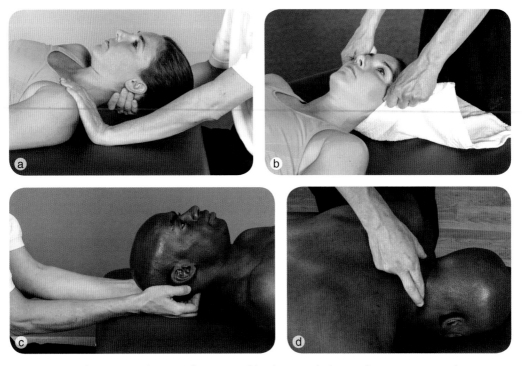

Figure 3.2 Therapist techniques for cervical lordosis include gentle, passive stretch to posterior neck tissues using (a) your hand, (b) a towel, (c) massage to the small neck extensor muscles and (d) gentle pressure to deactivate trigger points.

- Apply myofascial release techniques to the posterior neck. One technique is to place one hand beneath the occiput (as in figure 3.2a) and the palm of your opposite hand against the skin of the sternum and wait for the release, allowing your hands and the client's head to move as necessary.

- Teach your client how to stretch the muscles on the back of the neck.

- Teach your client how to perform active head and neck retractions.

- Test the strength of your client's neck flexors. If you find these to be weak, provide advice on appropriate strengthening. Poor endurance of the short cervical flexor muscles has been found in patients with increased cervical lordosis (Grimmer and Trott 1998); one way to test for this is to position your patient in the supine position and ask him to lift the head from the treatment couch. Most people are able to lift the head against gravity and retain the position, but a patient with weak neck flexors will find it difficult. Various approaches to assessment of these muscles have been put forward and reviewed by Jull and colleagues (2008).

- Advise your client on the correct sitting position for use of DSE equipment (see appendix), driving, reading, watching TV and so on.

- Address posture of the thoracolumbar region using the information in chapters 4 and 5. An increase in activation in cervical neck extensors has been found in slumped sitting, a position in which the pelvis is posteriorly rotated and the thorax relaxed whilst looking straight ahead (Caneiro et al. 2010). Increased activation of neck extensor muscles is detrimental to patients with increased cervical lordosis.

- Refer your client to a physiotherapist, osteopath or chiropractor when you think it is appropriate.

What Your Client Can Do

- Identify any activities that may contribute to the maintenance of a lordotic neck, and avoid these where possible. Not all of the contributing factors may be avoidable. For example, degeneration of the cervical spine could be a contributing factor that is unavoidable, whereas most people can correct poor neck posture when using a computer or driving.

- Correct neck posture when sitting or standing by paying particular attention to the spine. To counter the increased lordosis, it is helpful to give your client an image to help her visualize a lengthening of the neck. One such image is to imagine the body as a puppet with a string attached to the top of the head. When at rest, the puppet head may rest on the sternum or shoulders, squashed into the crumpled puppet body by gravity; when the puppet is in use and the string has tension, it pulls the head upwards and with it the neck, elevating the chest and lengthening the spine. The puppet arms might dangle downwards, depressing the shoulders and swinging at the puppet's sides. Similarly, clients can be encouraged to let their shoulders and arms relax, increasing the distance between the shoulders and head.

- Stretch the superficial muscles on the back of the neck. This could be as simple as performing neck flexion regularly. There are two ways to enhance this stretch.

Once in flexion, the client places one hand on the back of the head and applies very gentle overpressure. This facilitates an increase in range and stretches posterior neck tissues. However, this should be done with care because it places greater stress on upper cervical vertebrae and is contraindicated in clients with osteoporosis. It is a caution of clients with conditions affecting the vertebral artery. An alternative is to teach your clients to depress shoulders once in the position of flexion. Activation of shoulder depressors lengthens the upper fibres of trapezius and levator scapulae. Another way to stretch the muscles on the back of the neck is to rest with the head on a folded towel or a book (figure 3.3a). Once in this position, a client can use heels or buttocks to shuffle the body caudally, lengthening the neck as the head remains still.

- A client can stretch the deep neck extensor muscles by performing head and neck retractions. Ask your client to imagine the chin resting on a shelf and to slide the chin towards herself, avoiding head and neck extension (figure 3.3b). It is sometimes

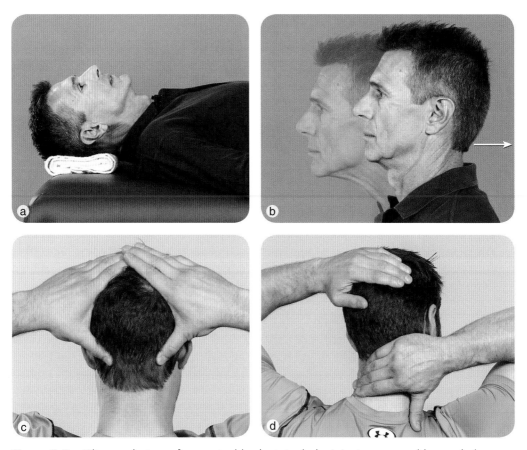

Figure 3.3 Client techniques for cervical lordosis include (a) using a towel beneath the occiput, (b) performing a head and neck retraction exercise, (c) identifying and massaging suboccipital muscles and (d) gently drawing the fingers across the neck combined with head and neck rotation to deliver a transverse stretch.

helpful to ask the client to face a mirror and to make a double chin, which is the same movement. If your client finds either of these movements difficult, position her supine, slide your finger beneath her neck and the treatment couch, and ask her to press the back of the neck into your finger. As your client does this, gently draw your finger away from the neck and towards the couch. This also encourages head and neck retraction. Note that when practicing retraction, some patients extend the head and neck. Extension is brought about by the very muscles you are encouraging your client to stretch and is therefore counterproductive. In the supine position a patient is more likely to perform the desired movement because extension is limited by the couch.

- Massage the back of the neck. Experimenting with ways to teach your client how to massage the back of the neck can help the client to identify the increase in tension here. Notice that if you place your thumbs beneath the occiput of your own skull (figure 3.3c), you can palpate the neck extensor muscles and can even feel these relax when neck retraction is performed, whereas if neck extension is performed, they contract. This position can therefore help you teach your client to identify whether he is performing neck retraction exercises correctly or simply as a means of massaging the suboccipital region. Gently pulling the fingertips across the neck can be combined with rotation of the head to facilitate a massage or stretch of tissues transversely. Try this for yourself: Place the fingers of your right hand behind your head on the left side of your neck, then draw them across the back of your neck, moving your fingers from left to right, as you turn your head to the right (figure 3.3d). This works because as you turn your head to the right, the back of your neck moves to the *left* and your fingers glide transversely across the skin. You can also use a therapy ball or tennis ball to gently compress and massage soft tissues.

- Strengthen neck flexors. One way to do this is to practice isometric neck flexion. Resting supine, your client simply lifts the head off the treatment couch in the same manner as would be used to test the strength of the neck flexor muscles. Breathing normally, the client attempts to hold the head off the couch for a count for five, thus performing an isometric contraction. Endurance can be built up daily and measured in seconds, with a client aiming to increase the time maintaining the position from 3 seconds to 7 seconds to 12 seconds, for example. This is quite effortful, and patients with hypertension should avoid this.

- Address thoracolumbar posture. Correcting poor posture in the thoracolumbar region—such as a slumped sitting posture—is likely to have a beneficial effect on the correction of neck posture.

Lateral Neck Flexion

A laterally flexed cervical spine may occur for several reasons. It could be habitual, due to a prolonged occupational or recreational posture. Or it could result from leg length discrepancy or scoliosis where lateral curvature of the spine in the thoracic region requires compensatory curvature to the opposite direction in the cervical spine. Lateral flexion can often be observed both posteriorly and anteriorly.

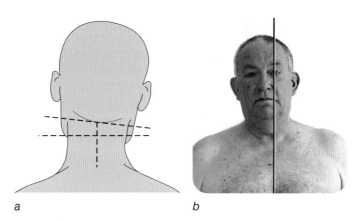

a   b

Figure 3.4 A laterally flexed cervical spine can be observed both *(a)* posteriorly and *(b)* anteriorly. This patient is laterally flexed to the right.

Consequences of Lateral Flexion

With lateral flexion, soft tissues on the side to which the head is laterally flexed are compressed, and those on the opposite side of the neck are lengthened. Intervertebral discs are compressed on the side to which the head is flexed to a greater extent than they are on the opposite side, as are facet joints. Prolonged compression of facet joints on one side of the neck could be detrimental to the functioning of these joints over time. The eyes are no longer parallel with the horizon, so there could be consequences for vision. With soft tissues spanning both the neck and shoulder, it is likely that, in time, such a posture will also adversely affect shoulder function.

TIP Observe the clavicles of a client with a laterally flexed neck. Usually the clavicle is raised on the side to which the neck is flexed. Treatment of soft tissues around the clavicle on that side could therefore be indicated.

What You Can Do as a Therapist

- Acknowledge that interventions may be limited where the lateral flexion is the result of leg length discrepancy, scoliosis or a laterally flexed thorax. If this is the case, your treatment may prove useful for decreasing symptoms such as pain but may not correct this neck posture.

- Help your client to identify the sorts of activities that could contribute to this posture. Often these are activities that involve elevation of the shoulder (on the side to which the neck is flexed), such as carrying a heavy bag on one shoulder, resting the arm (on the shortened side) on the window sill of a vehicle while driving or wearing

Table 3.2   Muscle Lengths Associated With Cervical Spine Laterally Flexed to Right

	Shortened muscles	Lengthened muscles
Area	Lateral neck flexors	Lateral neck flexors
Posteriorly	Right levator scapulae	Left levator scapulae
	Right upper fibres of trapezius	Left upper fibres of trapezius
Anteriorly	Right scalenes	Left scalenes
	Right sternocleidomastoid	Left sternocleidomastoid

an arm sling that is too short. Some people have a tendency to hold the head to one side when thinking or working.

- Help your client to compare how the left and right sides of the neck feel when gently stretched, and thus identify what tissues are tensioned more on one side than the other. There are two simple ways to do this. One way is to ask your client to adopt normal sitting posture and to relax the shoulders. As you gently depress one shoulder and then the other, ask your client to compare the sensation on each side. Although very little force is required to depress the shoulder in this manner, avoid this if your client has scoliosis or suffered a recent disc trauma, because either could be aggravated by unilateral pressure through the spine. The other method is to perform the same movements but with your client in the supine position: Squatting or kneeling at the head of the treatment couch, gently depress one shoulder and then the other (see the elevated scapula section, figure 9.11). In this position very little pressure is transmitted through the spine, and this position is therefore safe for most clients. Attuning oneself to the location of the tension in the neck is useful because it later helps a client monitor progress when performing stretches actively.

- Encourage your client to correct posture when sitting or standing. Once a client is aware that she holds the head laterally flexed, she can correct this posture.

- Passively stretch shortened tissues. You could begin by using either of the techniques described above to help your client compare the left and right sides of the neck, in sitting or supine positions, holding the end of range position for about 12 to 15 seconds. Or you could perform a passive-assisted stretch by applying gentle traction to the upper limb on the shortened side. Begin with your client resting with the head in a neutral position. Apply very slight traction to the shoulder on the side to which the neck is flexed, taking care to place your hands superior to the elbow joint. As you maintain this traction, ask your client to slowly perform lateral neck flexion away from you. In figure 3.5a the patient is being treated for flexion of her neck to the right. Or you could apply gentle overpressure to either the shoulder, or the head, or both, in either sitting (figure 3.5b) or supine positions.

- Apply soft tissue release on the shortened side, focusing on more specific structures—scalenes anteriorly and levator scapulae and trapezius posteriorly. For example, to stretch upper trapezius using this technique, gently depress the tissues on the side of the neck, taking care not to press too hard onto the clavicle or acromioclavicular joint. Some therapists use their fingers to depress the tissues; others use a forearm. Where tissues are pliable, other therapists prefer to gently grip the tissues. Once you have created a lock on the tissues, ask your client to flex the head to the opposite side, thus creating a gentle stretch (figure 3.5c).

■ Where you have identified scalenes to be palpably tight, the same technique can be used, gently fixing the tissues with one or two fingers on the concave side of the neck whilst your client is in the neutral position, and then asking the client to laterally flex to the opposite side. Some clients find lateral flexion difficult and may find it easier to rotate the head away from you.

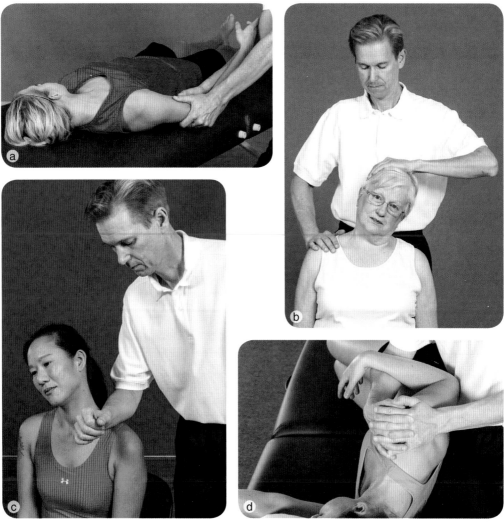

Figure 3.5 Therapist techniques for a laterally flexed cervical spine include (a) gentle passive traction of the glenohumeral joint combined with lateral neck flexion; (b) controlled, passive neck flexion with shoulder depression; (c) soft tissue release to shortened muscles; (d) passive stretch with your client in the side-lying position.

- Massage shortened tissues, in this case on the concave side of the neck in prone, supine or side-lying positions.

- Apply a passive stretch to the neck with your client in the side-lying position on the side to which the neck is flexed resting uppermost, the client's head resting on a pillow. Standing or kneeling by your client, cup your hands over the top of the client's shoulder and gently depress it. Avoid cupping your hands over the upper fibres of the trapezius of you can. As you gently pull the shoulder towards you, depressing it, the weight of the head prevents the head from moving and thus facilitates a controlled stretch to the soft tissues on the lateral side of the neck (figure 3.5d). If your client wishes for a greater stretch, do not use a pillow. Notice too how your client can localize the tissues in which she feels the stretch by altering the position of the head slightly, rotating it away from you, for example.

- Teach your client how to stretch the muscles on the side of the neck to which it is flexed.

- Use the myofascial release technique of a longitudinal arm pull on the side of the neck that is shortened (i.e., the side to which the neck is flexed).

- Test the strength of lateral neck flexors; if the flexors are weak, advise your client to consider strengthening these.

- Refer your client to a physiotherapist, osteopath or chiropractor where you think this is appropriate.

What Your Client Can Do

- Identify and avoid causal factors especially when carrying things or when sitting.

- Stretch shortened muscles. These are on the side to which the neck is flexed. To do this, the client simply performs lateral flexion to the opposite side. Applying gentle overpressure with one hand enhances this stretch, as does depressing the shoulder (figure 3.6a). Additionally, taking the arm behind the body is a variation of this stretch (figure 3.6b). Note that in this position some clients report feeling tension on the anterior neck, the consequence of tensioning anterior neck tissues by slight extension of the shoulder.

- If lateral flexors of the neck have been found to be weak, a simple way to strengthen these is to rest with the weaker side uppermost and simply lift the head from the floor, attempting to hold it in a neutral position. Each day the client could attempt to hold the head isometrically like this for a few more seconds until the client can retain this position equally well, whether resting on the left or the right side. Or, the client could simply perform isometric contraction of the lateral neck flexors by pressing against a hand whilst sitting or standing (figure 3.6c).

- Consider sleeping position. Sleeping on one side with the neck laterally flexed could also be a contributing factor to postural imbalance. Excessively thick or too many pillows leave soft tissues on the upper side of the neck in a shortened position and those on the mattress side of the neck in a lengthened position. Too thin or too few pillows leave soft tissues on the mattress side of the neck in a shortened position and those on the upper side of the neck lengthened. Filling the gap between shoulder and head correctly helps the neck remain in a more neutral, aligned position so that tissues are neither lengthened nor shortened on either side of the neck.

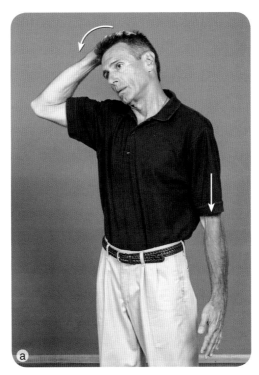

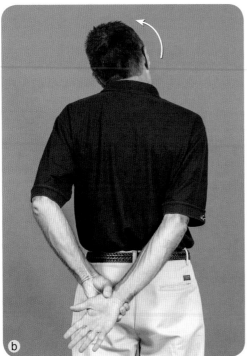

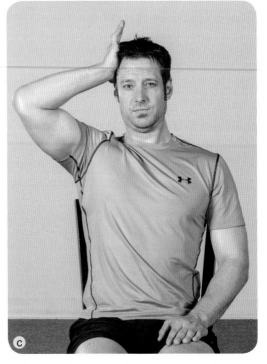

Figure 3.6 Client techniques for a laterally flexed cervical spine include *(a)* the application of gentle overpressure to the head or depression of the shoulder, which may be enhanced by *(b)* taking the arm on the side of the shortened muscles behind the body, plus *(c)* isometric exercises to strengthen lateral flexors where these have been found to be weak.

Forward Head Posture

In this posture the normal lordotic curve of the neck is lost and the cervical spine appears straight on x-ray. There is no definitive description for the forward head posture but, as the name suggests, it is one in which the head is observed to be forward (anterior) to the imaginary vertical line bisecting the body in the sagittal plane (figure 3.7b).

In measuring the relationship between the head, shoulders and thoracic spine, Raine and Twomey (1994) provide an illustration that helps in visualizing the forward head posture. In the sagittal plane, imagine a horizontal line passing through the tragus of the ear (this line happens to be called the Frankfurt plane) and another passing through the C7 disc. Then join C7 and the tragus. The adjoining line represents the relationship between the head and neck (figure 3.7a). Notice that as the head moves forward (anterior) with respect to the body, the angle formed between the C7 horizontal line and the adjoining line decreases (figure 3.7b).

To maintain the forward-looking position of the eye sockets, the head is tilted backwards on C1 and the atlanto-occipital region of the neck is considered to be hyperextended. The degree of extension is sometimes referred to as the excursion angle (figure 3.8). By superimposing this line on a photograph or when looking at your client, you can better judge whether the client has a forward head posture.

In rare cases the forward head posture is a controlled, temporary posture adopted by a patient to alleviate pain. An example of when this occurs is with cervicothoracic interspinous bursitis, perhaps as the result of prolonged extension of the head and neck, as might occur when looking up to paint a ceiling (Waldman 2008).

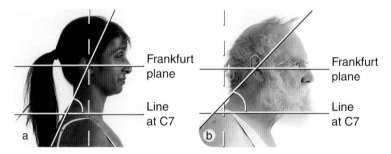

Figure 3.7 *(a)* Neutral head posture and *(b)* forward head posture with respect to the vertical line bisecting the body in the sagittal plane, showing a decrease in angle as the head moves anteriorly.

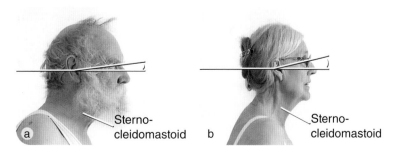

Figure 3.8 Excursion angles superimposed over these photographs with forward head posture reveal that *(a)* the male patient has a smaller excursion angle than *(b)* the female patient.

Consequences of a Forward Head Posture

There is a weakening of the deep cervical short flexor muscles. Grimmer and Trott (1998) found this to be true only for head-on-neck postures where there were large excursion angles in the upper cervical spine. As the head and neck move further into the forward head position, there is a tendency to extend the head, increasing the excursion angle. Such a posture lengthens the localized deep flexor muscles at that point, supporting the notion that they are weakened.

The female patient in figure 3.8b has a greater excursion angle than the male patient in figure 3.8a and is therefore more likely to have weaker deep neck flexors. This is evidenced by the hypertrophy of her sternocleidomastoid (SCM) muscle, which can be seen on the right side of her neck in the photo. Weakening of deep neck flexors is significant because these muscles also contribute to stabilization of the neck and provide proprioception. Not only is longus colli a flexor of the cervical spine, but the high number of muscle spindles it contains suggest that it is also important for proprioception. It is also a stabilizer of the neck during talking, coughing and swallowing. Consequences of weakness in longus colli are a decreased ability to flex the neck, especially against gravity (e.g., lifting the head from a pillow) and decreased stability of the neck during talking, coughing and swallowing. One might speculate that this would have a knock-on effect to jaw muscles and possibly contribute to temporomandibular problems.

There are other consequences of this posture. Scalenes may hypertrophy and spasm in the forward head posture, compressing the subclavian artery and vein and the ventral nerve roots of the C5-T1 spinal nerve as these pass between scalenus anterior and scalenus medial and above the first rib. Such compression results in pain and dysfunction that has been termed thoracic outlet syndrome. There is an additional effect on the sternocleidomastoid muscle. In order for SCM to flex the neck when working bilaterally, the synergists must stabilize the cervical spine. When this does not occur—as in the case of forward head posture and a weakening of longus colli and scalenes—bilateral contraction of SCM produces extension (rather than flexion) of the neck and an increase in the lordotic curve.

There is also increased activation in splenius capitis and trapezius in people with this posture (Noh et al. 2013), and this may be related to both pain in the neck and pain in the shoulder.

Finally, increased extension in upper cervical vertebrae may affect the muscles responsible for this movement, the suboccipitals. These are believed to contribute to proprioception, and a forward head posture may therefore have a negative effect on balance.

TIP Consider that this posture may be associated with repositioning of the mandible and an increase in activity of the muscles of mastication.

TIP Compression of nerves associated with C1 and C2 posteriorly (as in exaggerated excursion) could result in craniofacial pain.

Table 3.3 Muscle Lengths Associated With Forward Head Posture

Area	Shortened muscles	Lengthened muscles
Anterior neck	Longus capitis Longus colli Suprahyoid	Infrahyoid
Posterior neck	Suboccipitals	Levator scapulae

These muscles are shortened with the exception of their relationship to upper cervical vertebrae: The deep cervical flexors are lengthened where there is increased excursion in the upper cervical vertebrae.

What You Can Do as a Therapist

- Advise your client on corrective exercises to reposition the head. Look at figure 3.9 and consider the effect of sitting in a forward head posture. In each of the three siting positions, observe that the weight of the head is anterior to the vertebral column, but in figure 3.9c, the tendency to crane the head and neck forward is greatest. Observe your client sitting in the posture commonly adopted for work, driving or a seated hobby. How could the client be encouraged to sit in a more upright posture? One tip is to use a small cushion positioned at the lumbar spine. Notice that the thorax, and subsequently the head and neck, change position and are elevated when use of the cushion (or lumbar support) is inserted. You can try this for yourself. Sit slumped, taking note of your neck posture, and then place a cushion behind your low back. What has happened to the position of your neck? If you feel that how your client sits may be contributing to forward head posture, provide advice on the correct sitting position for use of DSE equipment (see appendix), driving, reading and watching TV.

- Massage shortened tissues, in this case the upper neck extensor muscles. This could be done in supine (figure 3.2c) or prone position. The supine position is useful because as you draw your hands from the base of the neck to the head, you can encourage your client to perform a gentle nodding movement. Resting with your fingertips at the base of the skull, this motion helps lengthen the short neck extensors

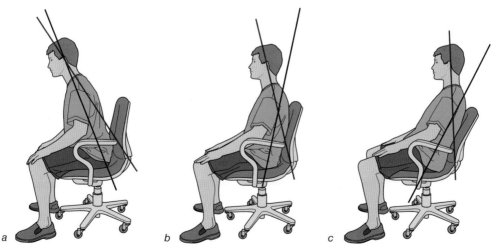

a b c

Figure 3.9 Sitting postures: *(a)* forced upright sitting; *(b)* neutral sitting; *(c)* slouched sitting.

and requires activation of the deep neck flexors, helping to strengthen these. Notice that this nodding movement is different from gross neck flexion.

In the prone position you can also encourage this gentle nod and stretch of posterior tissues by applying gentle traction to the base of the skull (figure 3.10a), although the nodding movement is more difficult for the client to perform. Asking your client to perform a chin tuck is one way to encourage contraction of deep neck flexors and a reduction in tone in upper neck extensors. The chin tuck position is especially useful when treating clients with increased adipose tissue on the back of the neck, where a lengthening of soft tissue can sometimes be difficult in the prone position.

- Treat any trigger points you find in suboccipitals and in other muscles. These may be addressed with gentle pressure (figure 3.2d)

- Teach your client how to stretch the muscles on the back of the neck.

- Teach your client how to perform active head and neck retractions (figure 3.3b).

- Test the strength of your client's neck flexors; if you find these to be weak, provide advice on appropriate strengthening. One way to test the strength of the neck flexors is to position your client in the supine position and ask him to lift the head from the treatment couch. Most people are able to lift the head against gravity in this manner. A patient with weak neck flexors will find it difficult to maintain a position of flexion. This is the craniocervical flexion test, which has had extensive research (e.g., Falla et al. 2004; Jull et al. 2008).

- Consider taping as a corrective device. It could be that the tension used with the application of tape will provide a mechanical effect preventing forward head posture and may be useful for patients who struggle with neck retraction exercises as a means of postural correction (Yoo 2013). Experiment with various taping designs, such as the shown in figure 3.10b.

- Address thoracic and lumbar postures because non-optimal thoracolumbar postures are associated with the forward heard posture.

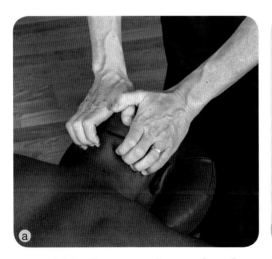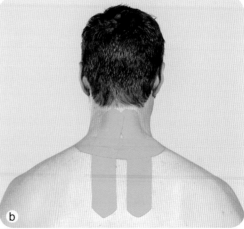

Figure 3.10 Therapist techniques for a forward head posture include (a) massage to short neck extensors in prone positions and (b) taping.

- Examine the muscles of mastication, such as temporalis, which may cause jaw and head pain due to hypertonicity.
- Refer your client to a physiotherapist, osteopath or chiropractor where you believe it is appropriate.

What Your Client Can Do

- Identify any factors that may contribute to the maintenance of a forward head posture and avoid these where possible. Pay particular attention to head and neck posture when using a computer, watching television or driving. Carrying a heavy backpack increases this posture (Chansirinukor et al. 2001), so avoid this.
- Correct the neck posture when sitting or standing. One way to visualize the strain a forward head posture places on the muscles on the back of the neck is to imagine that when is in the forward position, posterior neck muscles need to work like the reins of a horse to pull back the head over the torso. The further forward you hold your head, the more force is required to retain the position. A forward head posture is often associated with a kyphotic thorax. Avoiding a slouched position and paying attention to the position of the scapulae and thorax are likely to be a significant factor in correcting this posture. Sitting upright, retracting and depressing the shoulders, is a good starting point. For more suggestions on correction of a kyphotic posture, see that section in chapter 4.
- Stretch upper posterior neck tissues by resting with the head on a folded towel or a book (figure 3.3a). This is also a useful position in which to practice head retraction discussed in the next point.
- Stretch the deep neck extensor muscles whilst strengthening deep flexor muscles by learning to perform head and neck retractions. Gupta and colleagues (2013) suggest that this is more important in helping to correct the forward head posture than conventional isometric training. Ask your client to imagine the chin resting on a shelf and to slide the chin towards himself (figure 3.3b), avoiding head and neck extension. It is sometimes helpful to ask your client to face a mirror and to make a double chin, which is the same movement. If your client finds either of these movements difficult, position him supine, slide your finger beneath the neck and the treatment couch, and ask your client to press the back of the neck into your finger. As he does this, gently draw your finger away from the neck and towards the couch. This also encourages head and neck retraction. Note that when practicing retraction, some patients extend the head and neck. Extension is brought about by the very muscles you are encouraging your client to stretch and is therefore counterproductive. In the supine position a patient is more likely to perform the correct movement because extension of the neck is restricted by the couch.
- Strengthen global neck flexors. One way to do this is to practice isometric neck flexion. Resting supine, your client simply lifts the head off the treatment couch in the same manner as might be used to test the strength of the neck flexor muscles and holds the head off the couch for a count for five. Endurance can be built up daily and measured in seconds, with a patient aiming to improve the length of time in maintaining the position from 3 seconds to 7 seconds to 12 seconds, for example. Although it is not clear which exercises are best for the correction of cervical posture,

there is evidence to suggest that training of both the deep neck flexors (longus colli and longus capitis) as well as superficial flexors (sternocleidomastoid and scalenes) is useful in reducing neck pain (Falla 2004). If you believe that your client's pain results from poor cervical posture, neck strengthening exercises could be beneficial.

- Massage the suboccipital muscles. A way to do this is with the thumbs (figure 3.3c).

- As with an increase in the cervical lordosis, it is important to address thoraco-lumbar posture because this is likely to have a beneficial effect on the correction of the forward neck posture.

Rotation of the Head and Neck

When viewing a client from behind, you can sometimes observe more of the jaw on one side of the head than on the other. In this example the client demonstrates anticlockwise rotation (figure 3.11b). Rotation can be the result of many factors and may correspond with rotation in part of the thorax, rotation of a clavicle and protraction of a scapula.

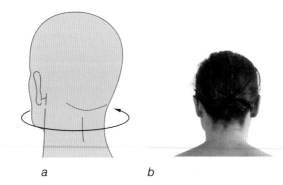

a   b

Figure 3.11   Anticlockwise rotation of the head.

TIP   Anticlockwise rotation of the head (to the left), for example, might correspond with ante-rior rotation of the right clavicle, posterior rotation of the left clavicle, anterior rotation of the second and third ribs on the right, but posterior rotation of the second and third rib on the left. There will be changes in the soft tissues associated with these bones and joints. This is just one example of a possible combination of factors, and every individual is unique.

What You Can Do as a Therapist

- Ask your client to perform rotations of the head in order to help identify tensioned tissues. One way to do this is to ask your client to look as far over each shoulder as she can and notice on which side she senses restriction. If when rotating to the right she feels restriction on the left of the neck, then it is to the right that she should practice stretching.

Consequences of Rotation

Rotation of the head tends to be minor and is perhaps least problematic of all head and neck postures. As with the other postures described in this book, there is a mechanical shortening of some muscles and a lengthening of others, as listed in table 3.4. The scalene muscles and the insertion of levator scapulae are often found to be sore on the side to which the head is rotated; sternocleidomastoid is often hypertonic on the contralateral side. Whilst the position of vascular structures changes with respect to one another in rotation of the head (Wang et al. 2006), this is unlikely to have any impact when the degree of rotation is minor, as described in this posture. The neck posture to which this section refers is different from what is apparent in cervical dystonia. Cervical dystonia can involve marked involuntary rotation of the head and requires specialist treatment. See National Institute of Neurological Disorders and Stroke (2014) for more information.

Table 3.4 Muscle Lengths Associated With Rotated Head and Neck

Area	Shortened muscles	Lengthened muscles
On rotation to the right (clockwise rotation)	Left sternocleidomastoid Left scalenes Right levator scapulae Right splenius capitis Right splenius cervicis	Right sternocleidomastoid Right scalenes Left levator scapulae Left splenius capitis Left splenius cervicis
On rotation to the left (anti-clockwise rotation)	Right sternocleidomastoid Right scalenes Left levator scapulae Left splenius capitis Left splenius cervicis	Left sternocleidomastoid Left scalenes Right levator scapulae Right splenius capitis Right splenius cervicis

Note that the degree of shortening or lengthening associated with this posture is minor.

- Encourage your client to correct posture, paying particular attention to any activities or positions that might contribute to rotation of the head. Clients with this posture are sometimes found to spend long periods using a computer or watching television where the monitor or TV screen is not central to the client's line of sight but positioned to one side. These clients may also be drivers who perpetually look over the same shoulder when reversing.

- Passively stretch shortened tissues using gross stretches. Use care when performing passive rotation of the neck toward the end of range, or where tissues feel tensioned. A safe stretch is to use a towel to gently roll the patient's head from left to right (figure 3.12a). The advantage of this technique is that it is less likely to result in overstretching of tissues because you as the therapist have less leverage when using a towel than when holding the head with the hands. Another advantage is that many clients relax the head and neck more readily than when you, the therapist, holds the head in the hands, perhaps because they can feel the treatment couch beneath their head, thus facilitating a stretch. Because this is a gross, rather than a specific, stretch, it does not necessarily target localized areas of tension. Use care when performing this movement on a client with Ménière's disease.

- Using table 3.4 as your guide, stretch specific areas of localized tension using massage, remembering to address cervical rotators on both on the posterior (figure 3.2*d*) and anterior (figure 3.12*b*) of the neck.

- Work to lengthen specific muscles using techniques such as soft tissue release. If working on the scalenes, gentle pressure using one or two fingers is all that is required to lock tissues before asking your client to slowly rotate the head to the opposite side (figure 3.12*c*). Shown here with a client seated, the technique is equally effective when performed with a client in the supine position. When working this region, avoid pressure to vascular structures—remove your finger if you feel a pulse. Notice that the stretch is enhanced if you apply traction to the skin by gently drawing your finger inferiorly before you ask your client to turn the head.

- Teach your client how to stretch the appropriate muscles. In this instance it is as simple as encouraging your client to perform active cervical rotation.

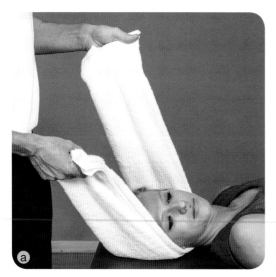

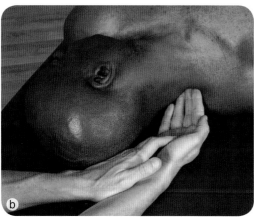

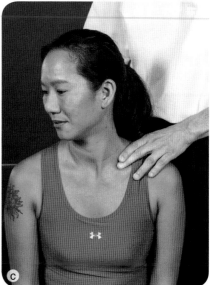

Figure 3.12 Therapist techniques for a rotated head posture include *(a)* passive stretches, *(b)* massage to cervical rotators on the anterior of the neck, and *(c)* specific stretches using techniques such as soft tissue release to, for example, scalenes where a gentle lock is applied to fibres and maintained as the client actively stretches the muscle.

- Refer your client to a physiotherapist, osteopath or chiropractor where you believe it is appropriate.

What Your Client Can Do

- Identify any factors that may contribute to the maintenance of a rotated head or neck and avoid these where possible. For example, be certain to centre work station equipment, alternate sides to which the head is rotated when reversing a vehicle and avoid sleeping face down with the head turned to the same side each night.

- Stretch neck rotators by performing rotation of the head and neck away from the side to which it is rotated. One way to encourage an increase in range is to ask your client to perform the stretch in the same seated position each day and to try to look further over the shoulder each day, observing what it is she can see when doing this. Another method is to suggest that the client add gentle overpressure using one hand (figure 3.13a), providing the client does not have any contraindications such as rheumatoid arthritis or cervical spondylosis.

- Adopt resting positions to counter the rotated posture. For example, if a patient is rotated anticlockwise (to the left), encourage the patient to rest with the head to the right, whether in prone or supine position. If resting supine, use a book or towel to help the client achieve a position of gentle neck traction at the same time (figure 3.13b).

- Once a client has felt soft tissue release to the anterior neck (figure 3.12c), she can learn to perform this technique herself.

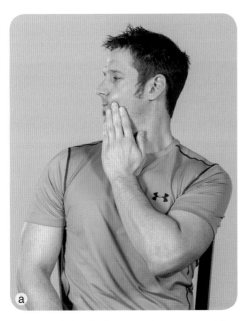
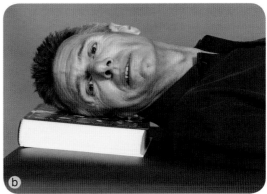

Figure 3.13 Techniques for a rotated head posture include (a) active stretches of the shortened tissues, perhaps with gentle overpressure; and (b) resting in postures that encourage these tissues to stretch, which may include using a book to help gentle traction of the neck at the same time.

Closing Remarks

In this chapter you learnt about four common neck postures: increased cervical lordosis, lateral neck flexion, forward head posture and rotation of the head and neck. The anatomical features of each are stated along with photographic examples and illustrations. The consequences of each posture are described, and for each pathology a table contains lists of shortened and lengthened muscles that can help plan your treatments. Treatment ideas are provided with suggestions about what you might do as a therapist and what your client might do to help correct each of the postures described.

Thoracic Spine

Learning Outcomes

After reading this chapter, you should be able to do the following:

- List three postures common to the thoracic region of the spine.
- Describe the anatomical features of each of these postures.
- Recognize these postures on a client.
- Give examples of the anatomical consequences of each posture.
- Name the muscles that are shortened and those that are lengthened in each posture.
- Give examples of appropriate treatments for the correction of each posture.
- Give the rationale for such treatments and, where relevant, state for which patients a particular treatment is contraindicated and why.
- Give examples of the kinds of stretches, exercises and activities that may be suitable for clients with specific postures of the thoracic spine and state for which clients these self-management tools might be contraindicated.

The three postures described in this chapter are kyphosis, flatback and rotated thorax. Viewed posteriorly, the thoracic spine is vertical. Viewed from the side, it is concave anteriorly and convex posteriorly. Together with the cervical and lumbar regions, this normal kyphosis improves the thoracic spine's resistance to axial compression. The centre of gravity of the head falls on the concave side of the thoracic spine, so it is no surprise that exaggeration of the curve posteriorly is a posture commonly seen in clinical practice. By contrast, loss of the curve, flatback in this region, is less common. It may be more common in patients who are hypermobile, where increased mobility of joints in the thorax permits a more upright posture than in the general population. Each of these postures may be associated with pain. In addition, the kyphotic posture is associated with abnormal shoulder mechanics and abnormal loading of intervertebral discs. A fourth posture, lateral curvature in the thoracic region, is covered in chapter 6, Scoliosis, because it is a complex posture associated with changes in other parts of the body.

Kyphosis

When a patient is observed to have an increase in the normal curve of the thoracic spine, the patient is described as having a kyphotic posture. Such a posture is most easily observed when viewing your client from the side. An overgrowth of fatty tissue in the cervicothoracic junction is often present, perhaps a response to this posture and the associated soft tissue imbalance. Kyphosis is a posture associated with aging and is frequently observed in elderly patients. There is a marked increase in the kyphotic angle after the fifth decade (O'Gorman and Jull 1987). Hyperkyphosis is a kyphotic angle greater than 40%. Health outcomes associated with this posture include thoracic back pain, restricted range of spinal motion, functional limitations, respiratory compromise and osteoporotic fractures (Greendale et. al. 2009).

The relationship between head position and the thorax has been investigated, and some researchers have found that as the head moves more anteriorly there is an increase in curvature from C7 to T6 (Raine and Twomey 1994). People who retain static work postures when seated at desks or when driving, or when carrying out tasks that encourage craning of the head, often portray kyphotic spines.

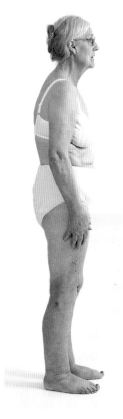

Figure 4.1 Kyphotic posture with an increase in the normal curve of the thoracic spine.

TIP In many cases of kyphosis there is also a forward head posture, so it is important to address the associated muscle imbalance. There may be internal rotation of the humerus, too, as scapulae protract and the humeral head changes its resting position within the glenoid fossa. For treatment ideas for these postures, see chapter 9.

Consequences of Kyphotic Posture

There is compression of the anterior longitudinal ligament and lengthening of the posterior longitudinal ligament and compression of the anterior aspect of intervertebral discs. Muscles and soft tissues on the back of the body (spinal extensors and the middle and lower fibres of trapezius) are lengthened, whilst those on the front of the body (pectorals and abdominals) are shortened. It has been postulated that the significant increase in load on the L5-S1 intervertebral disc could be a contributing factor in lumbar disc pathologies, progression of L5-S1 spondylolisthesis deformities and poor outcomes after surgery (Harrison et al. 2005). The increased activity in thoracic spine extensors could contribute to fatigue of these muscles and thoracic pain. This posture is likely to affect shoulder movement. For example, a large kyphosis has been associated with reduced arm elevation in older patients (Crawford and Jull 1993).

Table 4.1 Muscle Lengths Associated With a Kyphotic Posture

Shortened muscles	Lengthened muscles
Pectoralis major	Middle and lower fibres of trapezius
Pectoralis minor	Iliocostalis thoracis
Rectus abdominis	

Before treatment, note that caution is needed when attempting to address a kyphotic posture in certain client groups:

- Clients with or at risk of having osteoporosis (e.g., elderly or anorexic clients or clients *formerly* anorexic or bulimic). This is because some activities that encourage extension of the spine place stress on vertebrae and are therefore potentially harmful in patients with brittle bones.

- Clients who have recently had surgery to the chest or abdomen. Extension of the spine lengthens tissues on the anterior of the body and could affect wound healing.

- Clients whose postures are protective in nature, adopted consciously or unconsciously in response to emotional sensitivity (e.g., fear, anxiety, shyness, depression). Extension of the spine is a physical opening up of the anterior of the body and can leave some clients feeling emotionally exposed.

What You Can Do as a Therapist

- Acknowledge that interventions may be limited where the kyphosis is the result of degenerative changes rather than the poor posture associated with slumped positions.

- Help your client to identify causal factors and correct her own posture. The sorts of activities that could contribute to this posture are prolonged hunching when gardening, sitting at a desk, driving, rowing, playing computer games, and doing close work such as drawing, needlepoint or illustration.

- Passively stretch shortened tissues (in this instance, the pectorals). You could face the client to perform this stretch, or, for greater leverage, you could stand back to back, as in figure 4.2a. Take care not to overextend your client's spine; concentrate on extending the client's arms rather than arching the back. Spine extension is important, but trying to facilitate this whilst also stretching pectorals risks overstretching. One way to lessen the chances of this and to make the stretch more comfortable is to place a pillow behind the client. Take care not to overextend the shoulder.

- If stretching the tissues with the client in the supine position, adding a bolster or pillow positioned longitudinally against the thorax enables you to extend the shoulders slightly and thus facilitate a greater stretch for those clients for whom this is tolerable. Take care to also support the head and neck, as shown in figure 4.2b. If the bolster is too firm, it can be difficult for the client to remain resting on it comfortably because there is a tendency to roll to one side unless equal pressure is applied to both shoulders.

- When treating a client with a shoulder condition where depression of the affected shoulder could be uncomfortable or even contraindicated, the supine chest stretch

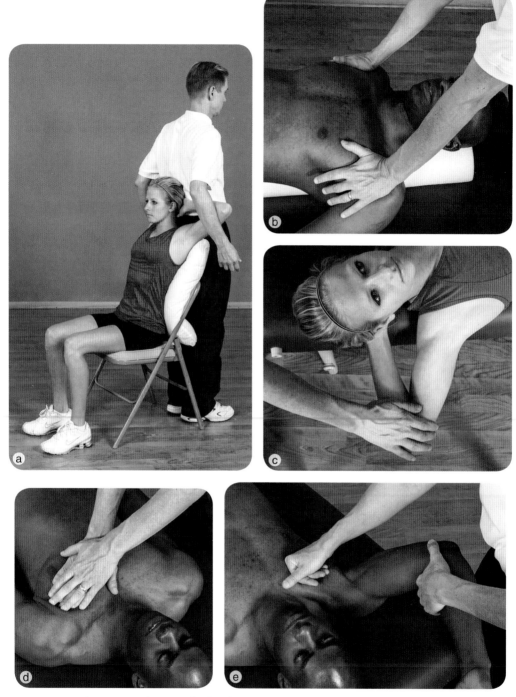

Figure 4.2 Therapist techniques for kyphotic posture include passively stretching pectoral muscles in (a) sitting or (b) supine positions, (c) passively stretching one side of the chest only, (d) massaging soft tissues of the chest and (e) applying soft tissue release to pectorals.

could be performed unilaterally. To do this, your client will need to be positioned diagonally across the treatment couch so that she can extend the shoulder on the side of the chest to be stretched. In this particular example the client has placed her hand behind her head, and you will discover that altering the position of the arm localizes the stretch to a different portion of the pectoral muscle (figure 4.2c).

■ Using the same positions that you use to stretch muscles passively, you could apply muscle energy technique.

■ Massage shortened tissues. Many clients feel comfortable with receiving massage to the clavicular portion of the pectoral muscle. The client can be supine, a position in which you have greatest leverage on this tissue. Where massage of the whole chest is acceptable, concentrate on stretching tissues from the sternum to the shoulder by using less of your massage medium than normal (figure 4.2d).

■ To enhance the stretch of chest tissues, you could use soft tissue release. Holding your client's arm so that the shoulder is flexed at about 90 degrees, lock the chest tissue using your fingers or fist, gently pushing the tissues away from you. Maintaining your pressure, slowly abduct your client's arm, passively stretching the tissues. See figure 4.2e, in which the therapist passively abducts the client's arm. This technique works equally well if the client abducts her own arm, moving it in such a way as to localize the stretch to different parts of the pectoral muscle by varying the degree of abduction.

■ Address alterations to the position of other upper-body parts that are associated with kyphotic posture, in this case forward head posture (chapter 3), protracted scapulae and internal rotation of the humerus (chapter 9).

■ Tape the upper back. One method shown to produce a decrease in thoracic kyphosis is that used by Lewis and colleagues (2005), described in the box that follows.

What Your Client Can Do

■ Identify any factors that may contribute to the maintenance of a kyphotic posture and avoid these where possible. Not all of the contributing factors may be avoidable. For example, where there are degenerative changes to vertebrae. Pay particular attention to posture when watching TV, and avoid slouching. Avoid hunching over a steering wheel or desk. When using a laptop position this to avoid a slouched posture and wherever possible use a detachable keyboard. Follow the advice for the correct set up of electronic display screen equipment (see appendix).

■ Actively stretch shortened muscles, in this case the pectorals. Contraction of the rhomboids (figure 4.4a) is a simple method of stretching pectorals and has the advantage that it can be performed surreptitiously almost anywhere.

■ Where chest stretches prove to be uncomfortable, a client could rest supine with a bolster or pillow placed longitudinally along the length of the thorax (figure 4.4b), allowing the arms to relax. As the scapulae relax into a neutral or retracted position, tissues of the anterior chest wall stretch. Clients with pronounced kyphosis may struggle to adopt this resting position and might even find it uncomfortable because it encourages both extension of the spine (from the normal or exaggerated

LEWIS TAPING TECHNIQUE

1. Demonstrate to your client how to extend the thoracic spine, and let him practice this a few times.

2. With the spine in extension, apply a strip of tape bilaterally from T1 to T12 (figure 4.3). Lewis and colleagues used Leukotape 1.5 inches (3.8 cm) wide.

3. Ask your client to fully retract and depress the scapulae and in this position apply the tape bilaterally from the centre of the spine of the scapulae to the spinous process of T12, thus forming a V shape (figure 4.3).

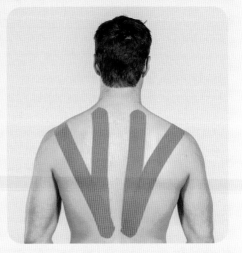

Figure 4.3 Thoracic taping. Tape strips applied bilaterally from T1 to T12 and from the centre of the spine of the scapula to T12 to form a V shape.

Lewis and colleagues made the important comment that whilst their taping protocol did extend the spine and retract, depress and posteriorly tilt the scapulae, in some patients this had a detrimental effect on shoulder range, supporting one of their conclusions, which was that mechanically correcting posture does not necessarily produce an improvement in function or a decrease in pain.

Consider whether, in the long term, it is better to encourage your clients to facilitate postural correction through strengthening of their own muscles than to encourage reliance on tape, the effects of which may be short lived. Teach your client exercises to strengthen weakened muscles using exercises such as the dart and prone rhomboid retraction to strengthen the middle and lower fibres of trapezius and thus help retract the scapulae.

kyphotic curve) and retraction of the scapulae. In such cases, simply resting supine in the floor will encourage correction of the spine, unless this is anatomically fixed.

- Some clients find it helpful to hold a small towel, thus stretching the anterior of the shoulder joint also (figure 4.4c).

- A wall or doorframe can facilitate a chest stretch where a client has a shoulder problem and cannot stretch both shoulders and both sides of the chest simultaneously. Try this for yourself. Notice that if you place your hand against a wall, elbow extended, and then turn your body away from the wall, the stretch can be localised to various regions of your chest when you raise your arm, sliding it up the wall before starting the stretch. Some clients find this too strong a stretch. Holding a vertical bar (rather than touching a wall) reduces the stretch because when holding a bar the

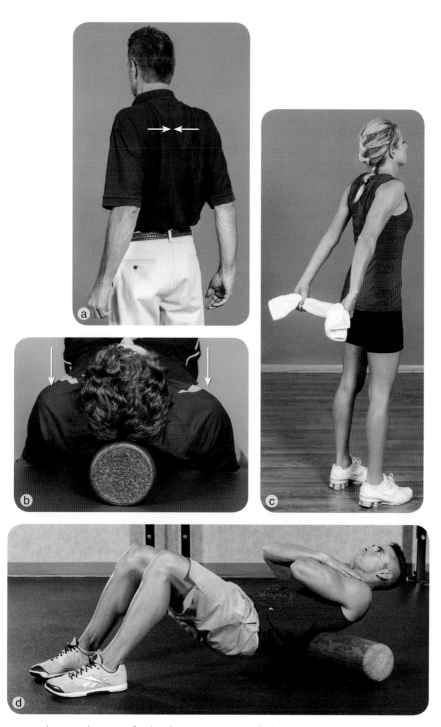

Figure 4.4 Client techniques for kyphotic posture include *(a)* stretching pectorals by contracting rhomboid muscles, *(b)* resting over a bolster, *(c)* using a towel, and *(d)* increasing thoracic extension by any means, including using a foam roller.

fingers are flexed and the wrist is more neutral, whereas with the palm against the wall the wrist and fingers are in extension.

- Strengthen the middle and lower fibres of the trapezius and the rhomboid muscles to help retract scapulae, using exercises such as the dart (see box) and prone rhomboid retraction. Aim to increase the duration the client can hold the position in each exercise pose. For prone rhomboid retraction, ask your client to rest face down and to abduct the arms to about 90 degrees. Next, ask him to gently lift the arms off the floor and supinate the forearm so that the thumbs are pointing upwards.

- Use a foam roller to facilitate spinal extension (figure 4.4d). Use extreme care because these rollers are made of firm Styrofoam; used in this manner, they place considerable pressure on individual vertebrae. This would be contraindicated for anyone with osteoporosis or a history of thoracic spinal pathology (such as joint subluxation or disc herniation). Clients with inflammatory conditions should use caution.

- Practice sitting up straight when performing seated tasks. It is not surprising that many people slouch, increasing the curve of the thoracic spine, because upright sitting requires more effort as evidenced by an increase in activation of thoracic spinal extensors compared to other seated postures (Caneiro et al. 2010).

- Address any cervical lordosis (chapter 3) and internal rotation of the humerus (chapter 9) if these areas of the client's body are affected.

- Performing yoga may help to correct kyphosis. Patients who adopt the mountain pose stance in yoga have been found to have a more correct stance, that is, a more symmetrical posture (in both frontal and transverse planes) than when in the relaxed stance. Not surprisingly, those who have been practicing for longer and more frequently demonstrate greater symmetry (Grabara and Szopa 2011). The mountain pose is one in which the patient attempts to elongate the spine in the sagittal plane, reducing the normal lumbar and kyphotic curves by engaging muscles to extend the spine vertically. The angle of kyphosis was reduced in patients aged 60 years and older with adult-onset hyperkyphosis (a kyphotic angle greater than 40 degrees) who took part in a 6-month study where they performed yoga for 1 hour 3 days per week for 24 weeks, compared to a control group (Greendale et al. 2009).

DART EXERCISE

1. With your client sitting or standing, locate the lower fibres of trapezius by palpating for the inferior angle of the scapulae and approximating the location of the lower fibres.

2. Ask your client to focus on this part of the back as you gently tap the fibres.

3. Then ask your client to gently retract and then depress the scapulae. Performing this in the prone position is more difficult because the scapulae have to retract against gravity.

Flatback

The term *flatback* usually describes a loss of the lordotic curve in the lumbar region. However, a reduction in the normal curve in the thorax can also sometimes be observed. This is difficult to illustrate photographically but presents as a flattening of the space between the medial borders of the scapulae, perhaps with less prominent spinous processes in the thoracic region (see figure 4.5).

In some cases a flattening of the thoracic region is the result of having had rods surgically inserted for the treatment of scoliosis. Rods used today are more flexible than earlier versions (called Harrington rods) that reduced lateral curvature but resulted in a loss of the thoracic curve in the sagittal plane and decreased strength and mobility in the spine. Advances in the treatment of scoliosis mean that a patient with rods in situ could have a more normal thoracic curve than a patient who had this same treat-

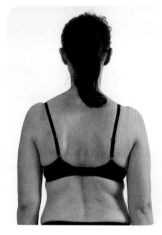

Figure 4.5   Flatback.

ment in the early 1960s when it was popular to insert rigid rods. However, Harrington rods are still used to fix spinal fractures (see Gertzbein et al. 1982), in which case the thorax may appear flat postoperatively, with decreased muscle mass, and the corrective techniques described here are likely to be ineffective.

Consequences of Thoracic Flatback

With this posture there is a lengthening of the anterior longitudinal ligament and a slackening of the posterior longitudinal ligament along with compression of intervertebral disc posteriorly. Given that both the discs and the longitudinal ligaments are important for providing stability to intervertebral joints, this is significant. Muscles on the anterior thorax are lengthened and those on the posterior are shortened. Hypermobile patients are often found to have loss of the normal kyphotic curve due to their ability to hyperextend the spine. Such patients appear to have good upright posture but often find standing erect painful and may flex the trunk slightly as a pain-avoidance posture. Thoracic flatback posture can be associated with pain in the thoracic spine perhaps because as a person stands increasingly erect, extending the spine, spinous processes start to approximate one another, compressing soft tissues.

TIP   Use caution when working with hypermobile clients. Whilst such clients may present with localized regions of tension in soft tissues, it is important to remember that they have excess laxity in joints that benefit from being made more stable through tightening rather than less stable through loosening. Whilst massage and soft tissue techniques may be beneficial as a means of pain management, it is important not to overwork any one region. Further, there is evidence to suggest that this group of patients may have lower bone density than the general population (Gulbahar et al. 2006) so localized deep static pressure to the spine should be avoided.

Table 4.2   Muscle Lengths Associated With Flatback

Shortened muscles	Lengthened muscles
Iliocostalis thoracis	Abdominals

What You Can Do as a Therapist

Whilst the techniques suggested here are helpful in reducing tension in iliocostalis and reducing pain, they will not alter a flatback posture in the thoracic region.

- Passively stretch shortened tissues, in this instance iliocostalis. To stretch this muscle a patient may simply flex forward, and most are able to do this without problems. Therefore, stretching tissues within specific regions of the thorax may be more beneficial. One way to do this is to apply an S-shaped stretch to soft tissues close to the midline. These are performed by using thumbs or fingertips to push the skin in opposite directions on each side of the spine (see figure 4.6a).

- Use soft tissue release to stretch iliocostalis with your client seated. Using fingertip pressure or knuckle pressure, gently lock the muscle and then ask your client to slowly flex the head and neck, thus bringing about a gentle stretch (see figure 4.6b).

- Massage iliocostalis with your client semi-seated. In this position the tissues are already in a lengthened position (see figure 4.6c). For clients who do not wish to be massaged whilst seated, the side-lying position can be used as an alternative because this enables a patient to flex the trunk slightly. In this position transverse strokes may be applied to iliocostalis.

- Gently rocking spinous processes can help relax soft tissues and provide pain relief. To do this, place your thumbs gently to the side of the spinous processes closest to you and apply gentle pressure in a rocking motion three or four times, working several times up and down one side of the thorax before repeating on the opposite side (see figure 4.6d).

What Your Client Can Do

- Avoid a military posture. Patients with thoracic pain often avoid standing erect because this aggravates their discomfort. Instead they have a tendency to adopt a slightly flexed spinal posture.

- Actively stretch iliocostalis. A popular stretch is the cat stretch used in yoga.

- Avoid sleeping on the front of the body because in this position gravity further extends the vertebral joints, decreasing (rather than increasing) the normal kyphotic curve.

- Consider general back strengthening. Exercise such as swimming is an excellent all-round conditioning and strengthening activity, and clients should be encouraged to experiment in order to determine which strokes are tolerable. If abdominals are

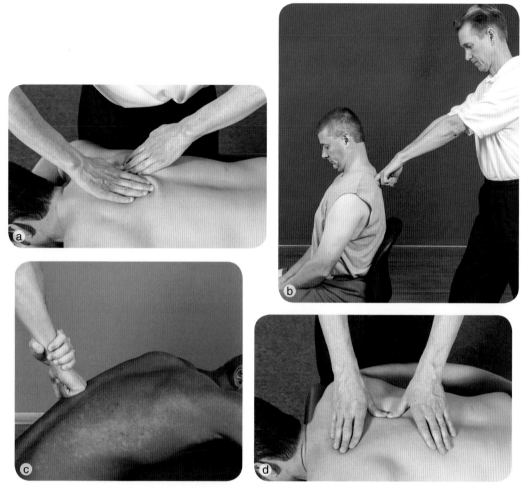

Figure 4.6 Therapist techniques for flatback posture include *(a)* localized stretches to paraspinal soft tissues, *(b)* soft tissue release with fingertip pressure gently locking the tissues as the client slowly flexes the head and neck, *(c)* massaging shortened iliocostalis in sitting and *(d)* applying transverse pressure to the spine and gently rocking spinous processes.

weak, regular abdominal strengthening could be considered. Whilst exercise for the back and abdomen will not change the thoracic flatback posture, it is important in maintaining strength of the spine and may lessen the likelihood of injury. Where a client with a flattened thoracic spine is known to be hypermobile, extra care is needed with the types of exercises undertaken.

Rotated Thorax

Rotation of the thorax is often noted when viewing a patient anteriorly or posteriorly where one side of the body appears closer to the examiner and one side further away. Posteriorly, it is often the shoulder blade that is prominent and alerts the observer to the possibility of thoracic rotation. With rotation of the thorax, not only is the scapula more prominent, the whole shoulder is closer to the examiner, as in figure 4.7b, which illustrates clockwise rotation. On an anterior view, you would expect this patient's *left* shoulder to appear closer to the examiner, perhaps with a more prominent left clavicle. Pronounced thoracic rotation is a feature of scoliosis, a posture covered in chapter 6. In this chapter the focus is on rotation of a more minor degree in patients who would not be deemed to have a scoliotic posture. Such posture could be the consequence of habitual rotation during a sporting activity—such as golf or one-sided rowing. Or, it might equally be found in those whose occupations involve repetitive or fixed rotation to one side, such as till operators at the check-out in a supermarket, or desk-based workers whose equipment is positioned to one side (e.g., a keyboard and computer screen in front of them but notepad to one side).

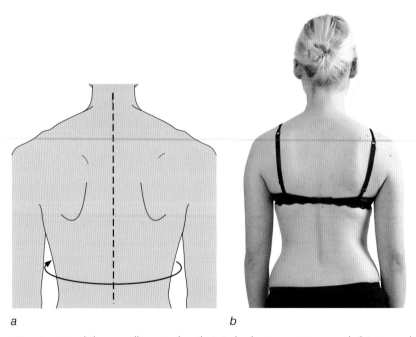

a   b

Figure 4.7 A rotated thorax, illustrated with *(a)* clockwise rotation and *(b)* viewed posteriorly with the patient's right shoulder appearing closer to the examiner than the left.

TIP Rotation of the thorax has a significant effect on the rest of the body, including the neck and lumbar spine, shoulders, pelvis, hips, knees, feet and ankles. Try rotating your thorax clockwise (to the right) and notice what happens to your left shoulder: It rotates clockwise and there is an increased likelihood of internal rotation of the humerus on the left shoulder. Notice also that even with mild clockwise rotation of a few degrees, to keep the eyes facing forwards, it is necessary to turn your head anticlockwise, contracting the muscles of anticlockwise cervical rotation.

Table 4.3   Muscle Lengths Associated With Rotated Thorax

Area	Shortened muscles	Lengthened muscles
Clockwise rotation	Deep thoracic spine rotators on the right Right internal oblique Left external oblique Left psoas Left lumbar erector spinae Muscles that rotate neck to the left	Deep thoracic spine rotator on the left Left internal oblique Right external oblique Right psoas Right lumbar erector spinae Muscles that rotate neck to the right
Anti-clockwise rotation	Deep thoracic spine rotator on the left Left internal oblique Right external oblique Right psoas Right lumbar erector spinae Muscles that rotate neck to the right	Deep thoracic spine rotators on the right Right internal oblique Left external oblique Left psoas Left lumbar erector spinae Muscles that rotate neck to the left

What You Can Do as a Therapist

- Appreciate that segments within the thorax can rotate to differing degrees, and patterns of activity between deep and superficial muscles vary within the thorax. For example, the action of multifidus may be to control motion at T5 and T8, and T11 may control coupling between rotation and lateral flexion movement (Lee et al. 2005). Global exercises to help strengthen weakened muscles and lengthen shortened ones may be useful, but for effective correction of posture in this region, it is likely that a physiotherapist or osteopath needs to conduct an assessment. Focused on mechanisms required for restoring normal function (rather than postural correction), Lee (2008) highlights the importance of specific assessment in this region of the spine.

- Help your client to identify and address causal factors. Are there any postures that involve rotation of the spine that the client maintains for prolonged periods?

- Passively stretch shortened tissues of the thorax by facilitating a gentle stretch to the direction opposite to that which your client is rotated. For example, if your client is rotated clockwise, stretch the torso in an anticlockwise direction. Instead of trying to rotate the thorax while stabilizing the pelvis, it is safer to stabilize the thorax and rotate the pelvis (figure 4.8a). Exercise care when performing passive stretches of the spine in this manner to avoid overstretching and potentially harming your client. Recognize that this is a global stretch and will not necessarily address localized points of soft tissue restriction.

- It may be useful to experiment with treatment positions. The stretch in figure 4.8b is commonly used to facilitate a stretch to the lateral side of the trunk and quadratus lumborum and could be useful in treating rotation.

- Massage shortened tissues of the trunk. Massage is a technique that specifically addresses shortened tissues of the trunk. For rotation to the right (clockwise), you will need to address the deep thoracic spine rotators on the right, the right internal oblique and the left external oblique. Rotators are located deep to back extensors.

Sometimes it is helpful to start by gliding down either side of the spinous processes using either your fist or forearm (figure 4.8c), assessing the tone of these muscles. You can then work in a more focused way using your fingers to palpate and massage specific areas of localized tension.

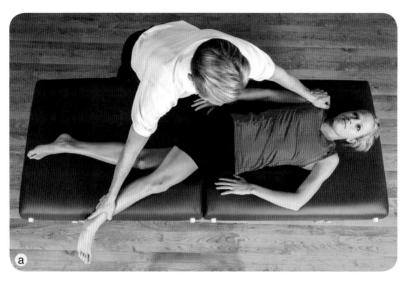

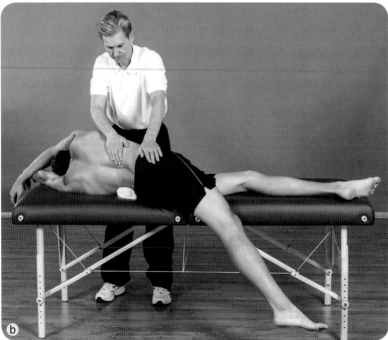

Figure 4.8   Therapist techniques for rotation of the thorax include *(a)* gentle passive rotation of the spine, *(b)* stretch to quadratus lumborum, experimenting with *(c)* side-lying positions or *(d)* the supine position to access the oblique muscles. *(continued)*

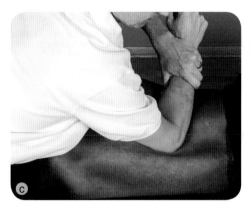 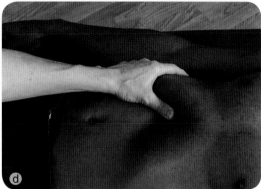

Figure 4.8 *(continued)*

- One way to access the obliques is to position your client on her side (figure 6.3*a*). This helps to open the area and, with the use of pillows, may be combined with slight rotation of the torso.

- When massaging obliques with your client in the supine position, take care not to press too hard beneath the ribs. Instead, experiment with asking your client first whether she can identify any tension in one side compared to the other side. Second, notice that when massaging this area, your client can facilitate a stretch. To do this, begin by gently pressing into the soft tissue as in figure 4.8*d* with the client's arm resting to one side. Then ask your client to raise her arm (on the side you are working) above the head, flexing at the shoulder until the arm is by the ear. This tenses the whole of the soft tissues on that side of the trunk, thus facilitating a stretch.

- Address shortness in other areas of the body. If you are treating rotation of the thorax to the right (clockwise rotation), you will need to assess and address psoas and lumbar erector spinae on the left and treat muscles that rotate the neck to the left.

What Your Client Can Do

- Identify and limit factors that may contribute to this posture. For example, ensure that a work station is set up correctly to avoid rotation to one side for prolonged periods. It is not always possible for athletes to address a preference for rotation to one side. For example, a golfer may not be able to swing the club equally well from one side as from the other; a javelin thrower will favour one arm; a canoeist may have a preference for using the paddle on one side over another. In such cases it may be necessary to address the imbalance through weight training, taking care to develop strength bilaterally (e.g., always performing the same number of oblique curls on each side of the body, always stretching both sides of the body for the same duration and to the same degree, taking note of where restrictions are felt in the body when stretching).

- Stretch the torso in the opposite direction to that which it is rotated. A simple stretch is to rest supine and twist the lumbar spine whilst keeping the shoulders on the floor (figure 4.9a). Clients will soon learn to which side they should rotate because that is the side to which they find most restriction.

- Seated stretches may be enhanced by holding a chair (figure 4.9b) to facilitate the stretch.

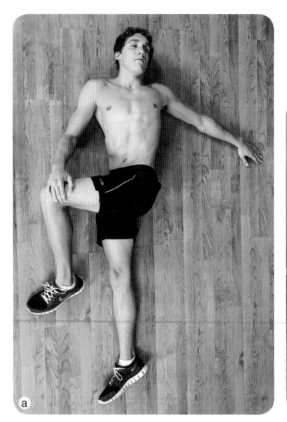
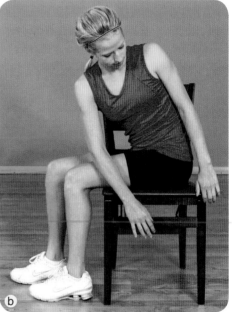

Figure 4.9 Client techniques for rotation of the thorax include stretches of the torso in (a) supine and (b) seated positions, using a chair to facilitate the stretch.

Closing Remarks

In this chapter you learnt about three common thoracic postures: kyphosis, thoracic flatback and rotated thorax. The anatomical features of each are stated along with photographic examples and illustrations. The consequences of each posture are described, and for each posture a table is provided with lists of shortened and lengthened muscles to help you plan your treatments. Treatment ideas are detailed with suggestions about what you might do as a therapist and what your client might do to help correct each of the postures described.

Lumbar Spine

Learning Outcomes

After reading this chapter, you should be able to do the following:

- List two postures common to the lumbar region of the spine.
- Describe the anatomical features of each of these postures.
- Recognize these postures on a client.
- Give examples of the anatomical consequences of each posture.
- Name the muscles that are shortened and those that are lengthened in each posture.
- Give examples of appropriate treatments for the correction of each posture.
- Give the rationale for such treatments and state for which clients a particular treatment is contraindicated and why.
- Give examples of the kinds of stretches, exercises and activities that may be suitable for clients with specific postures of the lumbar spine, and state for which clients these self-management tools might be contraindicated.

Viewed posteriorly, the lumbar spine is vertical. Viewed in the sagittal plane, it has a natural curve that is convex anteriorly and concave posteriorly. As with the cervical spine, this natural lordosis improves the lumbar spine's ability to withstand axial compression. But, unlike the cervical spine, the lumbar spine must support not only the head but also the entire torso and upper limbs and the forces associated with each.

The two postures described in this chapter are increased lordosis (hyperlordosis) and decreased lordosis (hypolordosis), popularly termed *flatback*. There are no widely accepted definitions for these postures. The lumbar curve is described as the angle between the superior end plate of the L1 vertebral body and the superior end plate of the sacrum. Factors such as age, sex, body mass index, occupation and sporting activity all affect this curve; therefore, it is difficult to establish what is a normal value. Some authors suggest that a lordotic angle of less than 23 degrees defines hypolordosis and an angle of more than 68 degrees defines hyperlordosis (Fernard and Fox 1985) when measuring this angle using roentgenograms (x-rays).

Been and Kalichman (2014) indicate this angle to be approximately 58.5 degrees and note that different curves can give the same angle, even when the same number of vertebrae are included in the calculation (not all researchers include all vertebrae in their measurements). Therapists are unlikely to have x-rays for the purposes of postural assessment, so these measurements are useful for the purposes of research but less helpful in a clinical setting. In practice it is more likely that you would use an inclinometer to measure lumbar lordosis and might record an inclinometer reading of less than −25 degrees as hyperlordosis and greater than −8 degrees to indicate hypolordosis (Scannell and McGill 2003). Topographic measurement of lumbar lordosis is often difficult because of variations in size, shape and orientation of spinous processes of lumbar vertebrae, paraspinal muscle tonicity and thickness of subcutaneous fat.

Ultimately, your desire to help correct a lumbar posture is likely to be because your clinical reasoning leads you to believe that by doing so you might help reduce a client's symptoms or because you think that creating postural change prophylactically would lessen the likelihood that your client will develop symptoms in the future rather than because you wish to help achieve a normal lordotic curve per se.

Increased Lordosis

An increased lumbar lordosis (hyperlordosis) can be best observed when viewing your client from the side. In the hyperlordotic posture the normal lumbar curve is exaggerated, hollowing the low back, and the pelvis is anteriorly tilted (see figure 5.1).

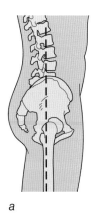 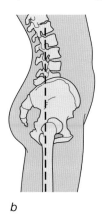 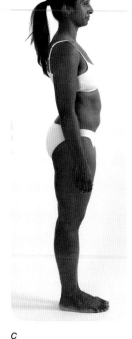

a b c

Figure 5.1 Lumbar spine indicating *(a)* normal lumbar posture, *(b)* increased lumbar lordosis and *(c)* hyperlordosis in a client.

Consequences of Increased Lumbar Lordosis

In this posture the posterior soft tissues of the lumbar spine are compressed; greater pressure is placed on the posterior aspect of intervertebral discs than on the anterior, affecting nutrient exchange (Adams and Hutton 1985); facet joints are subject to increased stress and a possibility of capsular strain (Scannell and McGill 2003). As with hyperlordosis in the cervical region, the posterior longitudinal ligament is compressed and the anterior longitudinal ligament lengthened, possibly affecting their stabilizing capabilities. Many clinicians theorize that factors associated with hyperlordosis contribute to osteoarthritis in facet joints in this region, degenerative changes in parts of the lumbar discs, low back pain and symptoms affecting the lower limb in some patients. There is currently no significant association between the lumbar angle and osteoarthritis, although having an increased lordosis angle is a risk factor for developing spondylolysis. The hyperlordotic spine is less able to withstand compressive stress, and patients with this posture may be at greater risk of injury when lifting heavy loads. Where hyperextension occurs in certain sports, this could be considered a risk factor for low back pain, such as during a golf swing (Hashimoto et al. 2013). Of course, a patient with a normal lumbar curve could also hyperextend the spine whilst playing sport but is less likely to do this than someone who already has hyperlordosis.

Several authors have looked at the effects of changing lumbopelvic posture on pelvic floor muscle activity and intravaginal pressure. As with much research, results were inconclusive. Capson and colleagues (2011) found that adopting hyper- or hypolordotic postures distorted pelvic floor muscles; hyperlordosis resulted in a stretch of these muscles and hypolordosis resulted in a shortening of the muscles. In the hyperlordotic posture there was lower force closure of the urethra and vagina, and the authors postulate that this has implications for patients with urinary incontinence. Similar research by Halski and colleagues (2014) did not support these findings.

Table 5.1 Muscle Lengths Associated With Increased Lumbar Lordosis

Shortened muscles	Lengthened muscles
Erector spinae group in the lumbar region	Abdominals
Psoas major	Hamstrings
	Gluteus maximus

Some studies suggest that lumbar lordosis increases with age (Tüzün et al. 1999) and is greater in some ethnic groups, but this is not conclusive. Researchers seem to agree that the curve increases with body mass index. The lumbar curve also naturally increases in late stages of pregnancy when a woman's centre of gravity changes due to the growing foetus and stretched abdominal muscles. It may also be exaggerated as the result of underlying pathology. For example, in the case of spondylolisthesis, one vertebra slips across another, sometimes resulting in a 'stepped' appearance in the lumbar region. Increased lumbar lordosis has been observed in athletes whose sports involve running, and this posture may be beneficial (Bloomfield et. al 1994).

TIP The imbalance between hip muscles associated with this posture could adversely affect hip function.

TIP There may be a shortening of the fascia in the region of the lumbar spine. Fascia of the lumbar spine is consistent with fascia both above and below it, spanning the upper and lower limbs. Shortening in one part is likely to affect function in areas removed from the lumbar spine itself.

What You Can Do as a Therapist

- Encourage your client to identify and avoid exaggerating the lumbar lordosis. Some clients know that they exaggerate this posture when standing, for example.

- Demonstrate to your client what a posterior pelvic tilt position feels like. Tilting the pelvis posteriorly lengthens lumbar erector spinae, but many patients struggle with knowing how to perform this simple manoeuvre. One way to demonstrate this exercise is to ask your client to help position a small towel beneath the low back and buttocks (see figure 5.2a). It is best if the towel is positioned high up in the lumbar region, around the T12-L1 area. Next, gently pull the towel from beneath your client using a series of short tugs. It is important that your client remain relaxed and not try to assist you by raising the buttocks off the couch. As the towel is tugged free, it gently moves the pelvis from its resting position to a neutral or posterior pelvic tilt position. In this way your client knows how this position feels and therefore has something to aim for when practicing pelvic tilts. Ask your client to notice how, in the posterior pelvic tilt position, the lumbar spine is flattened (perhaps touching the couch), and the abdominals are shortened.

- Lengthen shortened tissues with gentle passive stretches. A simple way to stretch the erector spinae of the lumbar region is to gently press your client's knees towards the chest, flexing your client's hips in the process. At the end of hip range you could apply gentle overpressure to stretch the lumbar spine. This stretch is difficult to perform when a patient has a large abdomen, because end of range cannot always be reached. You could facilitate a lumbar stretch further by holding the end position, or you could gently rock the lumbar region by moving very slightly in and out of the end of range. Some clients report feeling pinching or squashing on the anterior hip during this movement, perhaps as soft tissues are compressed. Where a client has osteoarthritis in one or both hips, use care; it may not be possible to gain a stretch at the end of range due to pressure on the hip. Flexion of the knees during this lumbar stretch would be contraindicated for a client with osteoarthritic or rheumatoid knees or swollen knees.

- An alternative position in which to apply a passive lumbar spine stretch is with your client in the foetal position (see figure 5.2b). Again, use caution when working with clients with hip or knee pathologies because of the degree of flexion required in those joints for this stretch. In this position you have good leverage and can apply pressure caudally, but you must also take care to safeguard your own posture.

- Massage extensors of the lumbar spine. In the prone position the lumbar lordosis can be exaggerated; for some clients this is uncomfortable during treatment. One solution that makes resting in the prone position more tolerable and enables better

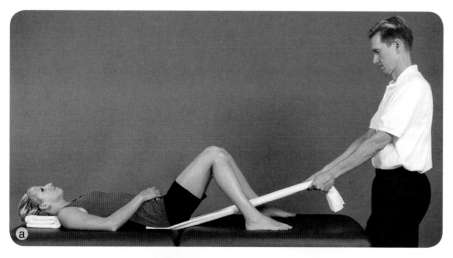

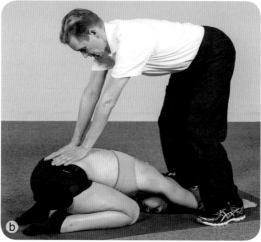

Figure 5.2 Therapist techniques for increased lumbar lordosis include *(a)* helping your client to achieve a posterior pelvic tilt position, and passively stretching shortened tissues by *(b)* applying a gentle stretch with your client in a foetal position.

access to the region is to offer your client a small cushion to place beneath the abdomen. In this manner the lumbar spine changes from extended to neutral and, with the cushion in place, lumbar erector spinae are slightly lengthened.

- Apply taping to inhibit anterior tilting of pelvis.

- Passively stretch psoas. The influence of psoas on the lumbar curve continues to be debated; some researchers argue that this muscle flattens the lumbar spine, and others state that as it contracts it pulls vertebral bodies anteriorly, exaggerating the lumbar curve. If on testing you have found psoas to be shortened, the stretches in chapter 7 for an anterior pelvic tilt will be useful.

- Use myofascial release techniques aimed to release the lumbar region, such as a cross-hand technique (figure 2.3) over the lumbar spine or a psoas release. For more information see Duncan (2014) and Earls and Myers (2010), respectively.

- Consider the posture of the thorax. Caneiro and colleagues (2010) found links between the thoracolumbar posture and the position of the head and neck. Harrison and colleagues (2005) concluded that with anterior translation of the thorax there are significant increases in loads and stresses on the lumbar spine and went so far as to say that the kyphotic posture could worsen an existing spondylolisthesis in the L5-S1 lumbar region. There is good rationale for addressing the entire spine when attempting to correct lumbar posture.

What Your Client Can Do

- Identify any activities that may be contribute to the maintenance of an increased lumbar lordosis and avoid these where possible. Not all of the contributing factors may be avoidable (pregnancy, for example). By contrast, patients *can* choose to avoid overly relaxed standing postures where the pelvis tilts anteriorly and the abdomen protrudes, thus increasing the lumbar curve, and can avoid sleeping on their stomach, another position that encourages lumbar lordosis. It is not only inactivity that can contribute to this posture. Sports which rely on strength in the hip flexor muscles could aggravate this posture, as psoas major pulls the lumbar vertebrae anteriorly (as many believe), increasing the lordosis. It has been postulated that wearing high heeled shoes increases lumbar lordosis but studies disagree as to whether this is the case, with some finding no exaggeration in lumbar posture in adults (Russell et al. 2012) and others concluding that wearing high heeled shoes can lead to lumbar hyperlordosis in adolescents (Silva et al. 2013).

- Frequently adopt resting positions in which the lumbar lordosis is decreased (flattened). Such positions can be achieved lying, sitting or standing. For example, resting supine with the knees and hips flexed, flexing the trunk whilst seated, and flexing the trunk whilst standing (see figures 5.3a-c). Even the slouched position, thought by many to represent poor sitting posture, causes the spine to flex, thus decreasing the lumbar curve. It may not be advisable to adopt this slouched position for prolonged periods of time, but it is an example of a resting posture that decreases the lumbar curve. Other positions that encourage flexion of the lumbar spine are sitting on a low chair or sitting on the floor with hips and knees bent (rather than outstretched). It seems reasonable to assume that the supine resting positions may be more effective at contributing to a change in the curvature of the lumbar lordosis than sitting or standing postures, as when supine the patient is most likely to relax.

- Actively stretch the lumbar spine. The aforementioned resting positions will all contribute to a lengthening of lumbar extensor muscles and relaxation of thoracolumbar fascia. One of the simplest ways to counter the hypolordotic position is for your client to rest on their side and bring their knees towards their chest, as far as is comfortable. If this is tolerable, they could rest on their back and hug both knees (figure 5.3d). The advantage of this position is that is focuses the stretch to the lumbar spine whilst the upper back and neck remain relaxed. Or, they could adopt a face-down foetal position as in figure 5.2b. In some cases, where the lordosis is

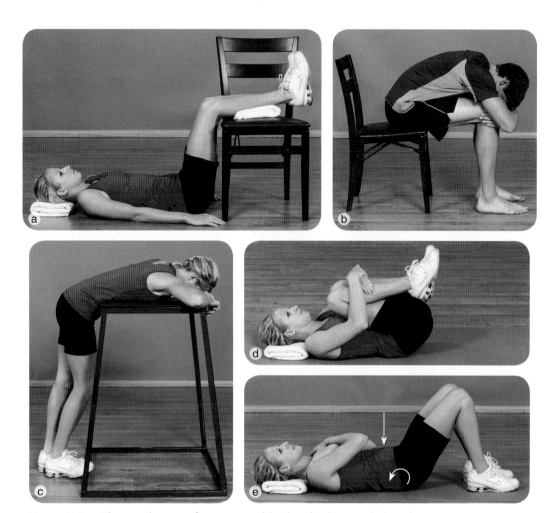

Figure 5.3 Client techniques for increased lumbar lordosis include adopting resting postures that temporarily decrease the lordosis such as *(a)* lying on the back with hips and knees flexed and supported; *(b)* resting in a forward flexed position whilst seated; and *(c)* resting in a supported, flexed posture whilst standing plus stretching the lumbar spine in positions such as *(d)* supine knee hugs and *(e)* posterior pelvic tilt.

particularly pronounced, it may be uncomfortable to attempt this stretch so a client could be instructed to attempt the resting positions first, gradually increasing their tolerance to a posture of increased lumbar flexion. By contrast, if your client feels that the aforementioned positions do not provide great enough stretch, she could sit on the floor with the knees bent, or on a chair, and place her head between her knees. In this position the spine is greatly flexed and, because considerable stress is placed on the anterior portion of lumbar discs, is contraindicated for anyone who has had disc problems.

■ After a series of experiments on the effect of posture on the lumbar spine, Adams and Hutton (1985) concluded that it might be advantageous to flatten the lumbar spine not only when lifting heavy weights but also when sitting. Practice posterior pelvic tilting in both standing and supine positions. This exercise changes the position of the pelvis and requires activation of lengthened, weakened muscles that are associated with an increased lumbar lordosis. To achieve the position, a patient must contract the abdominal and gluteal muscles simultaneously. It is a useful exercise for correction of the lumbar lordosis posture because, once a patient masters it, he or she can learn to correct the lordosis whilst sitting or standing. Instruct your client to lie on the floor with the hips and knees flexed and to place a hand beneath the back so that the palm is against the floor. Next, ask the patient to use his back to try to flatten the hand into the floor. To do this, the client will need to perform a posterior pelvic tilt (figure 5.3e). Teach this to your client in a seated position, you could ask him to place a hand behind his back, between the back and the back rest of their chair, and instruct him to press his hand against the back rest of the chair, again using his back to perform this manoeuvre.

■ Kendall and colleagues (1993) advocate that to correct excessive lumbar lordosis, this exercise is ultimately performed with the legs straight, a position that facilitates strengthening the abdominals at the same time. However, they point out that for some patients this can be difficult due to shortening of hip flexors, and they recommend the flexed hip position as a starting point for learning this important exercise.

■ Actively stretch psoas. Once a patient has mastered a posterior pelvic tilt, she is in a good position to stretch her psoas muscle in supine (figure 7.6a) or kneeling (figure 7.6b) positions. As with the passive stretch, if the patient adopts a posterior pelvic tilt whilst in either of these positions, it is more difficult for the lumbar spine to extend; the stretch is more effective and less likely to cause pain in the low back. Encourage your client to avoid flexing at the waist when kneeling because flexing decreases tension on psoas and reduces the effectiveness of the stretch. The kneeling position places considerable pressure on the patella, so clients with patellofemoral problems should avoid this position.

■ Finally, your client could wear a lumbar corset. Hashimoto and colleagues (2013) found that use of a lumbar corset in golfers reduced hyperextension of the lumbar spine. Their study investigated the value of a corset in the prevention of pain in this particular sport population by restricting *movement* of the spine rather than to correct a particular posture. Whilst physical immobilization in this manner decreases extension and is therefore beneficial as a temporary mechanism to prevent low back pain caused by hyperextension, the obvious disadvantage of using such a device purely to correct posture is that muscles associated with the lumbar spine will weaken. Hashimoto and colleagues also found that hip rotation in their patients increased and lumbar rotation decreased whilst wearing the corset. Use of a corset may therefore be beneficial for patients with discogenic problems but harmful for patients with osteoarthritis in the hip joint.

Decreased Lordosis

A decreased lumbar lordosis (hypolordosis) can be best observed when viewing your client from the side. In this posture the normal lumbar curve is lost, flattening the low back, and the pelvis is posteriorly tilted. As mentioned in previous chapters, this posture is sometimes referred to as flatback. A horizontal crease can sometimes be observed in the abdomen when viewing your client from the front. Such as crease can be seen on this patient even in the side view (figure 5.4).

There is a tendency for loss of lumbar lordosis in the elderly; as Sparrey and colleagues (2014) describe in their review, surgical management of lumbar posture restores posture at the expense of flexibility and has a high incidence of complications. Finding ways to help patients manage and possibly correct lumbar posture without the need for surgical intervention is likely to be beneficial.

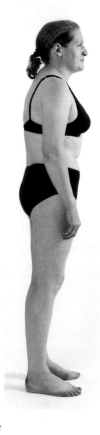

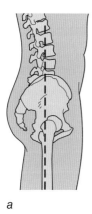
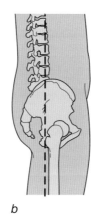

a   b   c

Figure 5.4 Lumbar spine indicating (a) normal lumbar posture, (b) decreased lumbar lordosis and (c) hypolordosis.

Consequences of Decreased Lumbar Lordosis

Although slight flexion of the lumbar spine reduces stress on the apophyseal joints (Adams and Hutton 1980) and compressive force on the posterior annulus, in the hypolordotic posture there is increased compressive stress on the anterior annulus of discs and increased hydrostatic pressure in the nucleus at low load levels (Adams and Hutton 1985). Whether pressure on the anterior portion of discs is harmful in the long term is likely to depend on the disc morphology of individual patients. Scannell and McGill (2003) note that a patient with a hypolordotic posture could be at greater risk for strain-related tissue failure than a person with hyperlordosis. Patients with low back pain often have hypolordosis, but it is not clear whether hypolordosis occurs before low back pain or whether these patients flatten their lumbar spines as a pain avoidance mechanism.

TIP The imbalance between hip muscles associated with this posture could adversely affect hip function.

Table 5.2   Muscle Lengths Associated With Decreased Lumbar Lordosis

Shortened muscles	Lengthened muscles
Lower abdominals	Lumbar erector spinae
Gluteus maximus	Hip flexors
Hamstrings	

What You Can Do as a Therapist

- Lengthen shortened muscles by applying passive stretches to gluteus maximus (figure 5.5*b*) and hamstrings (figure 5.5*a*). Lengthening of the hamstring muscles has long been advocated for the correction of hypolordosis (Kendall et al. 1993). In their study, Li and colleagues (1996) found no change in lumbopelvic posture after hamstring stretching, but others have questioned some of the methods used in that particular study (Gajdosik 1997). The hamstring stretch shown here is a good starting point for using muscle energy technique.

- Stretch and lengthen gluteal and hamstring muscles using deep tissue massage. When massaging hamstrings, you could apply strokes using your forearms (see figure 5.5*c*). You could also use soft tissue technique, locking tissues when they are in a shortened position before passively extending the knee.

- Treat trigger points in hamstrings and gluteals.

- In a study by Harrison and colleagues (2002) the application of passive lumbar extension traction increased the lordotic curve in a group of patients with low back pain who had reduced lumbar curves. One and a half years later the follow-up tests revealed that 34 of the 48 participants in the study had retained this improvement. The authors believe that the corresponding decrease in pain reported by patients was the result of the patients' changed lumbar posture. Whilst useful for research,

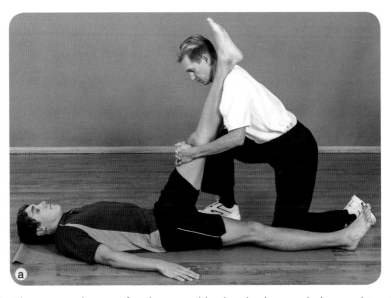

Figure 5.5   Therapist techniques for decreased lumbar lordosis include stretching *(a)* hamstrings and *(b)* gluteals and *(c)* massaging hamstrings. *(continued)*

the apparatus required to provide this traction was large and therefore not a practical treatment for use on a daily basis by most body workers.

- Tape the lumbar spine to encourage extension.

What Your Client Can Do

- Avoid prolonged postures that encourage lumbar flexion. For example, avoid slouched sitting or sitting on low chairs or the floor.

- Adopt resting postures that encourage extension of the spine. For example, sleeping on the front of the body and resting in the sphinx position (figure 5.6a), or resting on the back with a small firm pillow or a bolster beneath the lumbar spine, is a position similar (though less exaggerated) to the passive traction position used by Harrison and colleagues (2002), which the authors found decreased hypolordosis. Smith and Mell (1987) found that use of the sphinx position for 2 minutes a day for 4 weeks prevented a decrease in passive lumbar extension in male participants but not in females. Their participants were healthy and young, and it would be useful to replicate this experiment on patients with existing hypolordosis.

- Use of a lumbar support has been advocated to decrease hypolordosis in the sitting position (Majeske and Buchanan 1984). Many inexpensive versions of these are widely available and all similar. They are made of soft mesh or foam and attached to the back of a chair with elastic so that they can be moved up or down to suit the user's posture.

- Sitting with the chair seat inclined downwards at the front or sitting on a wedge-shaped cushion also increases the lumbar lordosis. It is not known whether the lumbar support, chair tilt position or use of a wedge will affect the posture of a patient with hypolordosis because these are believed to change spine posture in individuals with normal spines where range of motion is not impaired. However, such devices are worth considering as interventions for the purposes of experimentation.

- Actively practice extension of the spine. This could be as simple as leaning back whenever possible during the day.

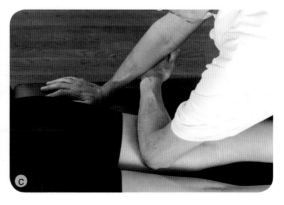

Figure 5.5 (continued)

- Certain physical activities encourage extension of the lumbar spine and could be incorporated into a weekly routine for patients with hypolordotic postures. For example, using a hula hoop requires both flexion and extension of the spine in order to keep the hoop in motion; swimming in the prone position encourages lumbar extension.

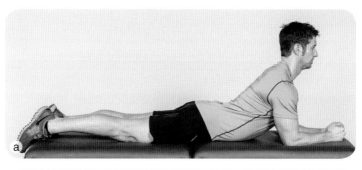

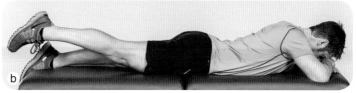

Figure 5.6 Client techniques for decreased lumbar lordosis include (a) resting in postures that encourage lumbar extension, such as the sphinx position, and (b) performing straight-leg hip extension in the prone position.

- Strengthen muscles that bring about an anterior pelvic tilt. A case study by Yoo (2013) describes how a patient with flatback was being treated for lumbar pain and given a 2-week programme of daily strengthening exercises for the erector spinae, iliopsoas and rectus femoris, and an increase in pelvic tilt angle was recorded after 2 weeks. Kendall and colleagues (1993) note that one of the challenges inherent to the correction of a hypolordosis is that gluteal muscles tend to be strong and hamstrings short in this posture, and exercises designed to increase lordosis when performed in the prone position activate these hip extensors. Kendall advocates increasing lordosis by raising the legs unilaterally in the prone position, extending the hip by only 10 degrees (figure 5.6b).

- Lengthen shortened muscles by doing active gluteal and hamstring stretches.

- Practice walking on an incline. Kim and Yoo (2014) found that in a study of eight participants with flatback syndrome, walking on a treadmill set to a 30-degree incline demonstrated a significant increase in anterior tilt of the pelvis after this activity. Although a protocol for duration and intensity is not established, this study is an example of a simple activity that could be adopted daily in order to determine its effect on hypolordosis.

Closing Remarks

In this chapter you learnt about two postures common to the lumbar spine: hyper- and hypolordosis. The anatomical features of each are discussed along with photographic examples and illustrations. The consequences of each posture are described along with a table listing shortened and lengthened muscles. Treatment ideas are provided with suggestions about what you might do as a therapist and what your client might do to help correct either of these postures.

6

Scoliosis

Learning Outcomes

After reading this chapter, you should be able to do the following:

- Define scoliosis of the spine.
- Describe types of scoliosis.
- Distinguish these postures on a client.
- Give examples of the consequences of scoliosis.
- Name the muscles that are shortened and those that are lengthened in this posture.
- Give examples of appropriate treatments for the correction of scoliosis.
- Give the rationale for such treatments and state for which clients a particular treatment is contraindicated and why.
- Give examples of the techniques that have been used in an attempt to correct scoliosis and state some of the advantages and disadvantages of the various techniques.
- State some of the non-surgical interventions for scoliosis and give examples of how a therapist or client can use these.

Scoliosis is a pronounced lateral curvature of the spine. Viewed posteriorly, the spine is vertical but in the scoliotic posture may appear to have an S or C shape, sometimes accompanied by severe thoracic kyphosis. There is a rib hump, where rotation of thoracic vertebrae cause ribs on the convex side of the curve to protrude posteriorly, and the skin is creased at the waist on the side of the concavity. Minor deviations of one or two vertebrae from the vertical position are common but do not constitute scoliosis. In true scoliosis there is marked asymmetry of the torso between the left and right sides of the body, anteriorly and posteriorly. Based on radiographs, a patient must have a Cobb angle of 10 degrees or more to be said to have scoliosis. As scoliosis becomes more pronounced, the Cobb angle increases (see figure 6.1).

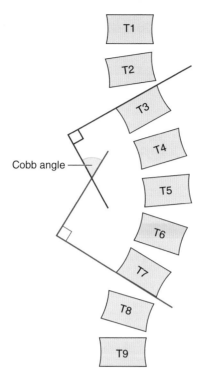

Figure 6.1   Cobb angle shown on scoliotic spines viewed posteriorly.

Compare the spines of patients *(a)* and *(b)* in figure 6.2, which both illustrate mild deviation of the spine from the vertical position, with an example of true scoliosis *(c)*. Patients in photographs *(a)* and *(b)* have spines that are convex on the left and concave on the right but would not be classified as scoliotic; the patient in *(c)* has a spine convex on the right and concave on the left and also shows marked kyphosis, a common feature of true scoliosis.

Types of Scoliosis

There are many ways to describe scoliosis—for example, whether it is functional or structural, whether it is congenital or acquired, by cause (for example, neuromuscular scoliosis), or by the age of onset (e.g., infantile, juvenile). Scoliosis is sometimes described according to the region of the spine that is affected. Following are the types of scoliosis:

- **Nonstructural scoliosis**. This could be thought of as functional scoliosis. There are no structural changes to vertebrae and no pathology affecting ligaments or muscles despite the spine appearing to deviate laterally. Causes include leg length discrepancy,

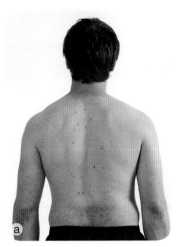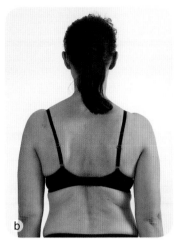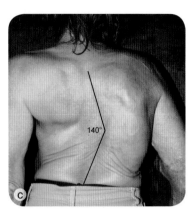

Figure 6.2 Lateral curvatures of the spine, presenting as convex on the left, with mild shift in torso to the left plus mild left-side rib hump *(a)*; convex on the left, with right-side skin crease at waist (b); and *(c)* convex on the right, with marked right-side kyphosis.

Photo c courtesy of Andrej Gogala.

impairment in vision or hearing, inflammation and muscle spasm. Nonstructural scoliosis disappears when the patient performs the Adam test and may be corrected by the patient without therapeutic intervention. This posture may be temporary. Nonstructural scoliosis, of which *(a)* and *(b)* in figure 6.2 are examples, has been disregarded clinically as being less important than structural scoliosis *(c)*. However, nonclinical scoliosis due to muscle imbalance may progress to structural scoliosis over time (Hawes and O'Brien 2006).

- **Transient structural scoliosis** is not permanent and can occur for many reasons, including muscle spasm, pain and disc herniation.

- **Structural scoliosis** involves changes to vertebrae that are both laterally flexed and rotated. Many categories are in this classification. Structural scoliosis does not disappear when the patient performs the Adam test and may not be corrected by the patient. It is caused by disease, injury or birth defect.

- **Idiopathic scoliosis** has no known cause. Around 80% of all cases of structural scoliosis fall within this category.

- **Congenital scoliosis** is structural scoliosis that is present at birth.

- **Acquired scoliosis** is structural and was not present at birth but occurs, for example, after vertebral fracture.

- **Neuromuscular scoliosis** is structural and related to a specific condition such as cerebral palsy, muscular dystrophy or poliomyelitis.

Consequences of Scoliosis

Pain is one of the main symptoms associated with this posture. Spinal nerves may be pinched where they exit the vertebral canal. Internal organs may become displaced, and theoretically their function could be compromised. Muscle imbalance and muscle fatigue are present. Spondylosis is also reported, and patients with true scoliosis may have shortness of breath due to asymmetry of the rib cage. There may be asymptomatic degeneration of intervertebral discs and facet joints. Additionally, the spine's ability to support the weight of the body is reduced, which can impair daily function. Because of the lateral shift in the torso, balance may be an issue. Patients with scoliosis many have concerns about body image and may have reduced self-esteem (National Scoliosis Foundation 2014). Weinstein and colleagues (1981) explain that for many years, studies perpetuated the idea that scoliosis led to severe disability and cardiopulmonary compromise, with mortality rates higher than in the general population. However, the grim prognosis regarding pulmonary function and risk of cardiac problems was not supported by one 50-year follow-up study (Weinstein et al. 2003).

Table 6.1 presents muscle lengths associated with an S-shaped scoliotic posture where the thoracic curve is concave on the left, combined with cervical and lumbar concavity on the right, as in figure 6.2c.

Table 6.1 Muscle Lengths Associated With Scoliotic Posture

	Shortened muscles	Lengthened muscles
Area	Concave side of the curve	Convex side of the curve
Neck	Right scalenes Right upper trapezial fibres Right levator scapulae Right cervical erector spinae	Left scalenes Left upper trapezial fibres Left levator scapulae Left cervical erector spinae
Thorax	Left intercostals Left thoracic erector spinae Left-side abdominals	Right intercostals Right thoracic erector spinae Right-side abdominals
Lumbar	Right quadratus lumborum Right lumbar erector spinae	Left quadratus lumborum Left lumbar erector spinae

TIP The muscles in table 6.1 are a generalization only. In all scoliotic postures there is a degree of rotation in vertebrae, and in many cases there is marked kyphosis. This will determine which muscles are shortened and which are lengthened, and you should assess these for yourself before treatment. For example, in figure 6.2 (b and c) the spine is convex on the right and left, respectively, but both have skin creases on the right, indicating shortening of the soft tissues in this region. As scoliotic postures involve rotation of vertebrae, length of the deep rotator muscles will be asymmetrical also. Imbalance between the upper and lower limbs is also common. Many therapists focus on the spine alone, but it is also important to address soft tissue shortening in other parts of the body.

Scoliosis

What You Can Do as a Therapist

- Refer to chapter 2, which begins with advice on describing postural observations. Sensitivity in the words you use is paramount and particularly important when treating clients with scoliosis who may have greater concerns regarding body image than other clients do.

- Recognize the limitations of hands-on therapies in the correction of this posture. Avoidance of factors likely to contribute to the posture has been advocated for correction of other postures in this book, but in 80% of scoliosis cases there is no known cause. Scoliosis is not the result of carrying something heavy, sleeping or standing postures, involvement in sports or minor discrepancy in leg length (Scoliosis Research Society 2015). It is therefore possible to advise your client on positions that might alleviate pain but not positions that will correct a scoliotic posture.

- Foremost, consider referring your client to a specialist for advice (e.g., the British Orthopaedic Association or the American Orthopaedic Association). The medical profession provides three main treatments for scoliosis (British Scoliosis Society 2008): observation (where the scoliotic curve is mild), bracing to prevent increases in the curve in more extreme postures and surgery to physically alter the shape of the spine. Non-surgical measures rarely control progressive scoliosis (Vialle et al. 2013). There is no evidence that physiotherapy, osteopathy, chiropractic, reflex-

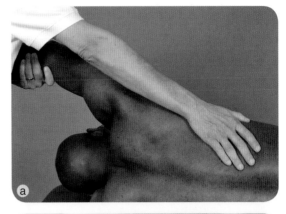

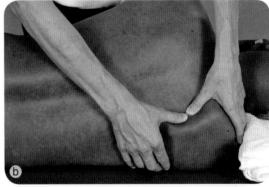

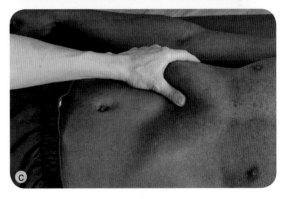

Figure 6.3 Possible techniques for addressing shortened muscles due to lateral flexion of the thorax to the right include *(a)* stretching with massage to the right latissimus dorsi in side-lying position, *(b)* stretching the right rhomboids and iliocostalis muscles and *(c)* gentle massage to the obliques.

ology or acupuncture can make a difference (Scoliosis Association [UK] 2014). However, in the case of mild idiopathic adolescent scoliosis it may be that physical exercise, tailored to the individual, prevents or reduces disability and facilitates a neutralization of the spinal curve (Negrini et al. 2001).

- Where the degree of curvature is low, activation of muscles may be effective at reducing the curvature of the spine (Curtin and Lowery 2014). It is vital to remember that strengthening of already shortened muscles, whether directly or indirectly, could worsen a scoliotic curve; for this reason, prescription and delivery of exercises should be undertaken only by professionals specialized in this field.

- Massage and stretch muscles on the concave side of the spinal curve. For example, with lengthened intercostals on the convex side of the thoracic curve and lengthened quadratus lumborum on the convex side of the lumbar curve, you will find shortened intercostals on the concave side of the thoracic curve and shortened quadratus lumborum on the concave side of the lumbar curve. Note in table 6.1 that muscles may also be shortened on one side of the neck or lumbar spine, and in all cases it is important to address shortened muscles on the anterior of the body as well as the posterior.

- Both for the comfort of your client and to facilitate access to shortened muscles, you might wish to experiment with varying the treatment position. For example, side lying can be useful for accessing latissimus dorsi and massaging intercostals and rhomboid and iliocostalis (see figures 6.3 *a* and *b*). If your client is comfortable in the supine position, remember also to address tension in abdominal muscles, again on the concave side of the curve (see figure 6.3*c*).

What Your Client Can Do

- Follow the advice offered by specialists. Having been a source of interest for many years, there is much evidence regarding treatment outcomes for the scoliotic posture and on which the medical profession can predict best outcomes. However, whilst surgery to correct scoliotic postures may alter the shape of the spine and may thus be said to have corrected this posture, it has high rates of post-operative complications. For example, in a review of 49 articles on the subject, Yadla and colleagues (2010) found that for 2,175 patients, there were 897 reported complications. So it is not surprising that many people with scoliosis look for alternative treatments. Solberg (2008) notes that in 1941 the American Orthopaedic Association concluded exercises should not be used in the treatment of scoliosis on the basis that studies showed exercise failed to halt the progress of the condition. However, Solberg explains that when methodological flaws were eliminated and the studies repeated, exercise *did* have a positive effect on scoliotic postures, arguing, 'Therapeutic exercise may actually produce improvement in the scoliosis and engender significant change both in body posture and in general functioning of the spinal column' (p. 107).

- Because of the variation in types of scoliosis and region of the spine affected, a specialist needs to prescribe corrective exercise, and organizations such as those listed are best suited to advise clients on accessing this kind of treatment. Figure

6.4 shows examples of the kinds of exercises such professionals might prescribe (in this example, for a thoracic spine that is concave on the left as in figure 6.2c). Movement may be brought about by more than one muscle group, and activation of an already shortened muscle could aggravate a scoliotic posture.

- Share information regarding the correction of the posture not only where the outcome has been positive but where an intervention has made no change. A good example of a self-reported case study is that presented by Gogala (2014), who details how a change in posture was achieved by wearing a corset, daily stretching of one side of the body, and carrying a backpack. He reports finding a hanging stretch particularly helpful as part of his routine to reduce his own scoliotic posture, and he advocates making a concerted effort to use the non-dominant hand. The uniqueness of individual scoliotic postures demands personalized programmes, and this means that the suggestions put forward by Gogala cannot be translated for use with anyone who has scoliosis. His case nevertheless is a valuable contribution to this subject matter.

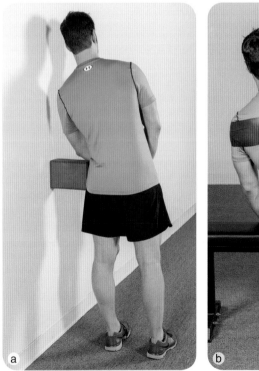
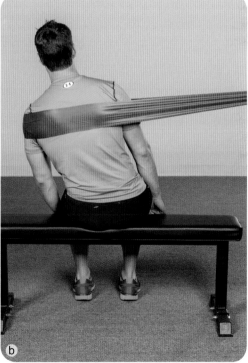

Figure 6.4 Exercises commonly prescribed for scoliotic posture include *(a)* using a wedge to block the left side of the pelvis as a patient attempts to shift the shoulders and torso to the left and *(b)* activating those same muscles by attempting to lengthen a stretchy band fixed around the left shoulder or torso.

- Rest in positions that lengthen and thus stretch shortened tissues. Specific resting positions will depend on individual postures and which muscles are shortened. For example, where shortened muscles are quadratus lumborum on the right and intercostals on the left (as in figure 6.2c), right-side lying over a rolled-up towel with the left arm abducted could prove useful.

- Participate in general exercise that strengthens both left and right sides of the body (such as swimming) rather than exercise that favours dominance of one side. Hurling, tennis and rowing are associated with a high incidence of scoliosis (Watson 1997), and lumbar scoliosis has been found in female dragon boat rowers (Pourbehzadi et al. 2012). Engagement in sporting activity used to be discouraged on the grounds that it might aggravate scoliotic postures. The stance of the National Scoliosis Foundation (2014) is that, whilst many scoliotic curves continue to increase with age, this does not seem to be related to sporting activity, and exercise in general is to be encouraged. Sports that involve extreme loading (such as in weightlifting) are potentially damaging (Gielen and Van den Eede 2008).

- Consider use of an orthotic, which may correct nonstructural scoliosis that is due to a leg length discrepancy (Hawes and O'Brien 2006).

Closing Remarks

In this chapter you have learnt to define and describe scoliosis and are provided with examples of mild, nonstructural scoliosis as well as one of severe structural scoliosis. The consequences of scoliosis are discussed plus the muscles that are shortened and those that are lengthened in this posture. Being a complex, three-dimensional posture, scoliosis requires specialist intervention, but now you have examples of the kinds of treatments you could provide as a therapist and the sorts of things you could advise a client about. Although the treatments you can provide for scoliosis are more limited than those for the postures described in chapters 3, 4 and 5, the information presented in this chapter should enhance your understanding of what can and cannot be done to correct this posture.

Correcting the Pelvis and Lower Limb

In part III you will learn about 4 postures specific to the pelvis and 10 postures that may be observed in the lower limb. The postures covered in chapter 7, Pelvis, are anterior pelvic tilt, posterior pelvic tilt, pelvic rotation and laterally tilted pelvis. Chapter 8, Lower Limb, includes internal rotation of the femur, genu recurvatum (knee hyperextension), genu flexum (flexed knee), genu varum (bowlegs), genu valgum (knock knees), tibial torsion, pes planus (flatfoot), pes caves (high arch), pes valgus (pronated foot) and pes varus (supinated foot).

Pelvis

Learning Outcomes

After reading this chapter, you should be able to do the following:

- List four postures common to the pelvis.
- Describe the anatomical features of each of these postures.
- Recognize these postures on a client.
- Give examples of the anatomical consequences of each posture.
- Name the muscles that are shortened and those that are lengthened in each posture.
- Give examples of appropriate treatments for the correction of each posture.
- Give the rationale for such treatments and state for which clients a particular treatment is contraindicated and why.
- Give examples of the kinds of stretches, exercises and activities that may be suitable for clients with specific postures of the pelvis and state for which clients these self-management tools might be contraindicated.

The four postures described in this chapter are anterior pelvic tilt, posterior pelvic tilt, laterally tilted pelvis and rotated pelvis. In this chapter, these postures are considered in isolation but are frequently observed in combination (e.g., where the pelvis is tilted anteriorly and rotated).

The pelvis supports the weight of the axial skeleton and upper limbs and transmits forces from these into the lower limbs. It also transmits ground forces up through the lower limbs to the spine. In each case, forces pass through the sacroiliac joint (SIJ), supported by sacroiliac ligaments acting as shock absorbers. The spine, pelvis and hip joints are inherently linked: Movement in any one affects the other two. Perhaps it is because of this and its dual force-transmitting function that some therapists believe the position of the pelvis is fundamental to overall posture and that, to bring about postural change in any part of the body, assessment and (if necessary) correction of pelvic position is crucial.

Figure 7.1 illustrates how, in the neutral pelvic position, there is general symmetry in the coronal plane: The left and right iliac crests are level, as are the posterior superior iliac spines (PSIS) and ischia (see figure 7.1a). In the sagittal plane, the anterior superior iliac spines are approximately parallel with the pubic bones (see figure 7.1b). In the transverse plane, neither the left nor right side of the pelvis is more prominent when viewed either anteriorly or posteriorly (see figure 7.1c).

Postural assessment of the pelvis is based on the assumption that the right and left sides of the pelvis are mirror images of one another. However, when 71 variables (such as bone thicknesses, distances between bones and angles between bones) were compared on a set of anatomical specimens, Boulay and colleagues (2006) found significant asymmetry in seven of the variables. They noted that there was a kind of spiraling of the entire pelvis; the upper part (the iliac blades) rotated clockwise and the lower part (the pubic symphysis) rotated anticlockwise (figure 7.2). (Their results indicated rotation was unidirectional.)

Boulay and colleagues believe this asymmetry is due to forces induced through walking (i.e., clockwise torsion of the pelvis is induced by the upper-body movement and anticlockwise torsion is induced by lower-limb movement). The reason for unidirectional rotation is that walking cannot be considered a symmetrical activity: Clockwise rotation could be because the dominant lower limb has a greater role in propulsion than the non-dominant one, and in right-handed individuals—the majority of the population—anticlockwise rotation of the lower part of the pelvis could be induced by the dominance of right hip propulsion over left hip propulsion. This information suggests

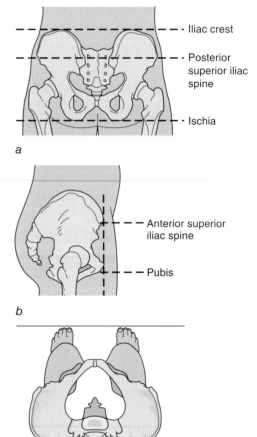

Figure 7.1   The neutral pelvic position viewed from the (a) posterior, (b) sagittal and (c) transverse planes.

that unless a patient is ambidextrous, there will always be a natural asymmetry to the pelvis in the transverse plane, something to consider when performing postural assessment. Caution is also required when planning corrective treatment of pelvic posture. Gnat and colleagues (2009) used a series of exercises that induced asymmetry in healthy adults, demonstrating that the presence of an asymmetrical pelvis does not necessarily indicate an underlying pathology. As with other postures in this book, you may wish to consider whether it is necessary to attempt to correct an asymmetrical pelvic posture. An anteriorly or posteriorly tilted posture corresponds with an imbalance in flexor and extensor muscles.

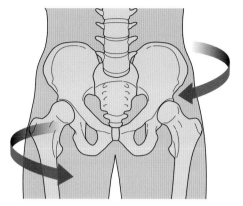

Figure 7.2 Boulay and colleagues' spiraling of the pelvis. The lumbar spine and bones of the hip retain proper alignment, while the top part of the pelvis rotates in one direction and the lower half in another.

Anterior Pelvic Tilt

In this posture the anterior superior iliac spine (ASIS) falls anterior to the pubic bones in the sagittal plane (figure 7.3b) unlike in the neutral pelvic posture when these points are aligned (figure 7.3a). Notice how when observing a client with this posture the waistband of the underwear sometimes provides a clue to pelvic position (figure 7.3c). With the lower limb fixed, anterior tilt of the pelvis produces hip flexion and corresponds with an increase in the lumbar curve.

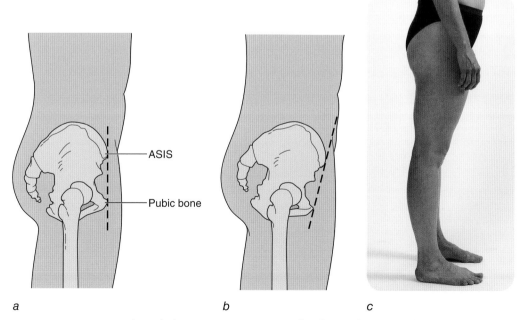

ASIS

Pubic bone

a   b   c

Figure 7.3 Anterior pelvic tilt demonstrating (a) neutral pelvis with ASIS and pubic bones in alignment, (b) anterior pelvic tilt where the ASIS and pubic bones are no longer in vertical alignment and (c) patient with anterior pelvic tilt and characteristic sloped appearance of underwear.

Consequences of Anterior Pelvic Tilt

The position of the sacrum is associated with various degrees of spinal curvature, as is the shape of the SIJ auricular facet (Kapandji 2008). Compared with the position of the sacrum associated with a more neutral spine shape, where there is an increased curvature (and associated anterior pelvic tilt), the position of the sacrum becomes more horizontally orientated. This in itself may be of little consequence. However, the shape of the auricular facet has been found to vary among sacra associated with different spinal shapes, and it seems reasonable to assume that the shape of this facet suits that particular spinal shape with which it is associated. Could changing the orientation of the pelvis (and sacrum) from a neutral position to an anterior pelvic tilt have a detrimental effect on sacroiliac joint function by reducing the ability of this joint to withstand forces?

Nutation and counternutation are movements of the sacrum about an axis with respect to the ilia. (There is debate about where the axis of rotation lies.) With anterior pelvic tilt (red arrows in figure 7.4) the sacrum moves in the opposite direction (blue arrows in figure 7.4), a movement that has been termed *counternutation*. Looking at figure 7.4, consider the position in which the spine would move if there was no counternutation of the sacrum: Fixed at its base to the first sacral bone, the lumbar spine (and all of the vertebrae above it) would be forced forward, away from the vertical position. Counternutation is important because it marginally decreases the degree to which the spine has to right itself back to vertical.

Where anterior pelvic tilt is pronounced or prolonged, could the sacrum be forced into counternutation in order for the spine to remain in a vertical position? What consequence might this have for the SIJ? Although the degree of SIJ movement is considered small (1-3 mm) (Brunstromm 2012), many therapists attribute back pain to dysfunction in this joint. Also, the sacral ligaments are strong and counter both nutation and counternutation. But could prolonged anterior rotation of the pelvis

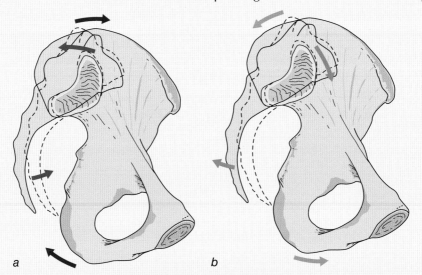

a   *b*

Figure 7.4 Counternutation *(a)* and nutation *(b)* of the sacrum seen in the anterior pelvic tilt and posterior pelvic tilt conditions, respectively.

ANTERIOR PELVIC TILT

stress the ligaments responsible for checking such movement, perhaps even affecting those muscles associated with these ligaments (e.g., the superior tendon of biceps brachii and the sacrotuberous ligament)?

Anterior movement of the acetabulae over the heads of the femurs changes the point of contact between these bony surfaces, the consequences of which are not known. Additionally, increased hip flexion corresponds with increased torques of the medial rotators of the hip and decreased torques of the lateral rotators. This could also affect the position of the femoral head in the acetabulum and the area of the head of the femur and acetabulum through which weight bearing and ground reaction forces are transmitted, and theoretically could lead to degenerative changes and adversely affect hip function in the long term.

An anteriorly tilted posture corresponds with an imbalance in flexor and extensor muscles (see table 7.1), which could adversely affect hip function. Finally, this posture corresponds with an increase in the lumbar curve and shares the consequences of that posture: As the pelvis tilts anteriorly, soft tissues of the posterior lumbar spine are compressed and greater pressure is placed on the posterior aspect of intervertebral discs than on the anterior, affecting nutrient exchange (Adams and Hutton 1985); facet joints are subject to increased stress and there is a possibility of capsular strain (Scannell and McGill 2003). Imbalance between longitudinal ligaments of the lumbar spine could alter their stabilizing capabilities; an anteriorly tilted pelvis could predispose a patient to osteoarthritis in lumbar facet joints, degenerative changes in parts of the lumbar discs and low back pain; it can also give rise to symptoms affecting the lower limbs.

Table 7.1 Muscle Lengths Associated With Anteriorly Tilted Pelvis

Area	Shortened muscles	Lengthened muscles
Torso	Lumbar erector spinae Psoas major	Rectus abdominis
Hip	Rectus femoris Iliacus Tensor fasciae latae Sartorius	Gluteus maximus Hamstrings

TIP Where there is anterior tilt of the pelvis with increased lumbar lordosis, there is also likely to be an increase in the thoracic and cervical curves, and these should be addressed also.

What You Can Do as a Therapist

Because this posture corresponds with that for increased lumbar lordosis, the treatment options are the same. Rather than repeat these, they are listed here along with the corresponding figure references in the section on increased lumbar lordosis in chapter 5, in which you can find more detailed descriptions.

- Note that this posture may be advantageous for participation in sports that involve running (Bloomfield et al. 1994), and you should consider whether correction will be beneficial.

- Encourage your client to identify those times when he stands with an anteriorly tilted pelvis and avoid this posture where possible. For example, when standing while tired, some clients relax into the anterior tilt posture.

- Teach your client how to perform a posterior pelvic tilt using the description for figure 5.2a. When taught correctly, a patient can learn to voluntarily rotate the pelvis posteriorly to such an extent as to significantly decrease the lumbar curve (Day et al. 1984). It is believed that proper pelvic alignment is important to dancers, for example, for the efficient execution of certain movements such as external rotation of the hip along with effective muscle recruitment. One method of teaching posterior pelvic tilt is to describe it as tucking the tailbone under (Deckert 2009).

- Passively stretch the lumbar extensor muscles using the suggestions provided for figure 5.2.

- Massage the lumbar spine using the suggestions provided in chapter 5.

- Tape the pelvis into a more neutral position. Taping the pelvis into a posterior pelvic tilt position decreased SIJ pain in a group of women who habitually wore high-heeled shoes (Lee et al. 2014). Although this study was an attempt to decrease pain, if taping is effective in pelvic realignment it could be considered as a temporary measure to help your clients learn what a more neutral pelvic posture feels like.

- Passively stretch psoas using the suggestions provided in chapter 5.

- Massage rectus femoris. The aim is to stretch this muscle using deep massage strokes from the distal to proximal ends of the muscle.

- Stretch rectus femoris. This can be performed supine (figure 7.5a) or prone (figure 7.5b). Stretching the rectus femoris muscle in a prone position could be harmful if the client has a history of trauma to the low back because the lumbar spine extends in this position. One way to overcome lumbar extension is for your client to perform a posterior pelvic tilt whilst you retain the position of the leg, thus performing the stretch herself without your needing to flex the knee further. This is also a good starting position for using MET. An alternative is to place your hand on the pelvis before flexing the knee, preventing movement in the pelvis and spine. Placing a rolled-up towel or bolster beneath the knee takes the hip into extension and facilitates a greater stretch of anterior thigh tissues.

- Use soft tissue release to iliacus. It is interesting to note that, with no other intervention, when STR is applied to iliacus, both active and passive hip extension appears to increase. To use this technique, gently lock anterior hip tissues with the hip in passive flexion (figure 7.5c) and maintain this as your client extends the hip (figure 7.5d). Be wary of pressing too deeply too soon; get feedback throughout the procedure.

- Use myofascial release techniques specifically on the lumbar region and psoas.

What Your Client Can Do

- Learn to maintain a more neutral pelvic position when standing. Regularly performing a posterior pelvic tilt will increase the endurance of gluteal and abdominal muscles and help counter an anteriorly tilted pelvic position. Instructions on performing a posterior pelvic tilt are in the suggestions provided for figure 5.2a.

- Strengthen abdominal, gluteal and hamstring muscles. Because these are the muscles used to tilt the pelvis posteriorly, it seems reasonable to attempt to strengthen

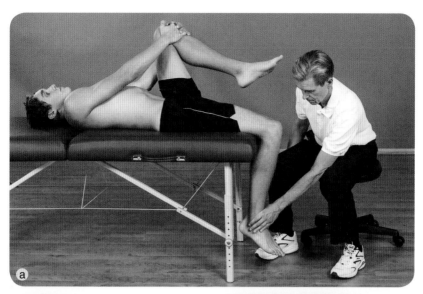

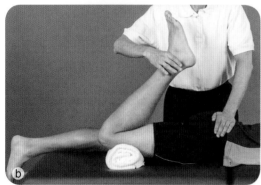

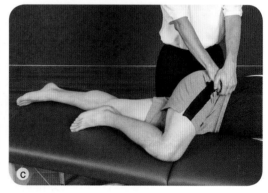

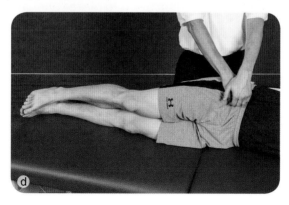

Figure 7.5 Therapist techniques for an anteriorly tilted pelvis include stretching rectus femoris in (a) supine and (b) prone positions and applying soft tissue release by (c) locking iliacus and maintaining the lock as your client (d) extends the hip during the stretch.

and shorten them. Abdominals will be strengthened by performing the posterior pelvic tilt.

- Stretch the muscles of the lumbar spine. There are many ways to do this. Examples are in figures 5.3a-e.

- Stretch hip flexors using stretches such as those in figures 7.6a and b. Performing a posterior pelvic tilt once in the stretch position increases the stretch. Stretching the psoas in the supine position can cause the client to extend the spine, increasing rather than decreasing the lumbar lordosis during the stretch. To overcome this, encourage your client to posteriorly tilt the pelvis as they practice this stretch.

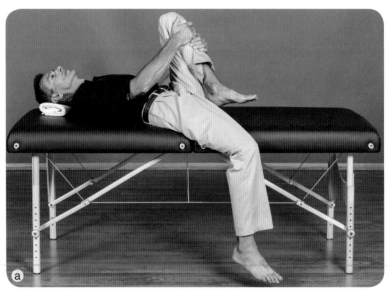

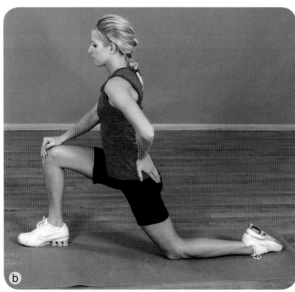

Figure 7.6 Stretches for hip flexors for patients with anterior pelvic tilt include *(a)* in the supine position with the leg hanging over a bed or couch and *(b)* kneeling.

Posterior Pelvic Tilt

In this posture the ASIS falls posterior to the pubic bones in the sagittal plane (figure 7.7b) unlike in the neutral posture where these points are aligned vertically (figure 7.7a). With the lower limb fixed, posterior tilt of the pelvis produces hip extension and corresponds with a decrease in the lumbar curve. There is sometimes tension in the abdominal muscles, which may be observed by an increased transverse abdominal crease (figure 7.7c).

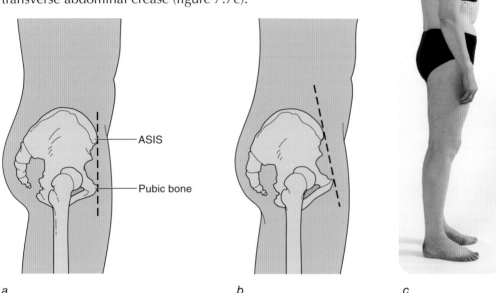

a   b   c

Figure 7.7 (a) Neutral posterior pelvic tilt, (b) posterior pelvic tilt with ASIS posterior to the pubic bones, (c) patient with posterior pelvic tilt.

TIP Where there is tension in abdominal muscles, it can pull on anterior fascia, depressing the rib cage and hampering thoracic extension.

What You Can Do as a Therapist

This posture corresponds with that for decreased lumbar lordosis, and the treatment options are the same. The options are listed here along with the corresponding references to figures in which you can find more detailed descriptions.

- Lengthen shortened muscles by applying passive stretches to gluteus maximus and hamstrings (figure 5.5a, b). The hamstrings and pelvis are inherently linked. Passive movement of the lower limb in straight-leg raising induces pelvic movement almost immediately, within only about 9 degrees of leg movement (Bohannon et al. 1985). Attaching to the ischia, hamstrings pull on the pelvis, bringing about a posterior pelvic tilt when they contract. Shortened hamstrings could contribute to the retention of this posture. Static stretching of the hamstrings permits greater pelvic tilt and lumbar flexion when activities requiring lumbar flexion are performed (López-Miñarro et al. 2012) but it is not known whether static stretching of the hamstrings would ultimately affect pelvic posture in the sagittal plane. Any effects may be temporary.

Consequences of a Posteriorly Tilted Pelvis

Compared to a neutral pelvis, as the pelvis tilts posteriorly, the sacrum becomes more vertical and the coccygeal bones fall closer to vertical. Unless there is a significant change in pelvic tilt when seated, a patient with a posteriorly tilted pelvis could have coccygeal pain when sitting for prolonged periods.

With posterior tilt of the pelvis, the sacrum is forced into nutation (see figure 7.4b) in order for the spine to remain in a vertical position. As with the opposite posture, anterior pelvic tilt, changing the position of the sacroiliac joint (SIJ), and the way it transmits forces from the ground and lower limbs to the spine, and from the torso and upper limbs to the legs, could be detrimental to the functioning of this joint.

A posteriorly tilted posture corresponds with an imbalance in flexor and extensor muscles (see table 7.2), which could adversely affect hip function. As with hypolordosis of the lumbar spine, there is increased compressive stress on the anterior annulus of discs and increased hydrostatic pressure in the nucleus at low load levels (Adams and Hutton 1985).

Table 7.2   Muscle Lengths Associated With Posteriorly Tilted Pelvis

Area	Shortened muscles	Lengthened muscles
Torso	Lower abdominals Gluteus maximus	Lumbar erector spinae Psoas
Hip	Hamstrings	Iliacus Rectus femoris

- Stretch and lengthen gluteal and hamstring muscles using deep tissue massage (figure 5.5c).

- Treat trigger points in hamstrings and gluteals.

- It is difficult to tape a posteriorly tilted pelvis into a more neutral position. This is because there are no discernable bony points on which to anchor your tape on the distal posterior pelvis. One option is to encourage your client to adopt a neutral pelvic position by performing an anterior pelvic tilt, then to tape the skin of the lumbar spine in this position. This will not fix the pelvis in an anterior—or even in a neutral—position, but will alert your client to changes in the pelvis as the adoption of a posterior pelvic tilt begins to traction the tape.

What Your Client Can Do

- Avoid prolonged postures that encourage a posterior pelvic tilt. For example, avoid slouched sitting or sitting on low chairs or the floor.

- Adopt resting postures that encourage extension of the spine (figure 5.6a).

- Use a lumbar support when sitting.

- Sitting with the chair seat inclined downwards at the front or sitting on a wedge-shaped cushion increases anterior pelvic tilt.

- Practice exercises that mobilize the lumbar spine and therefore encourage movement in the pelvis, including movement from a posterior pelvic position to a more neutral position.

- Strengthen muscles that bring about an anterior pelvic tilt: erector spinae, iliopsoas and rectus femoris. See figure 5.6*b* for an exercise suggested by Kendall and colleagues (1993).
- Lengthen shortened muscles by doing active gluteal and hamstring stretches.
- Practice anterior pelvic tilts. These are the opposite action to posterior pelvic tilts.
- Practice walking on an incline.

Pelvic Rotation

Pelvic rotation occurs around a vertical axis in the transverse plane. This may be observed as one side of the pelvis being closer to the examiner than the other, irrespective of whether the patient is viewed from the front or the back. The vertical axis may be the center of the pelvis (when a patient is weight bearing through both feet) but is more commonly the hip (coxal) joint of the supporting leg in single-leg stance, as occurs during walking (Levangie and Norkin 2001).

The terms used to describe the direction of rotation vary according to the axis point. When the vertical axis is at the center of the pelvic rotation, it may be described as being clockwise (forward rotation of the left ilium) or anticlockwise (forward rotation of the right ilium). This is evidenced by one side of the pelvis appearing closer to the examiner than the other, and it is exaggerated for the purposes of illustration here (figure 7.8). For example, when viewing a patient anteriorly, an observation that the patient's left ilium is closer to the examiner (figure 7.8*a*) indicates that the pelvis is rotated clockwise. Correspondingly, when viewed posteriorly, the right ilium of this patient would appear closer to the examiner (figure 7.8*b*). Conversely, an observation that the right ilium is closer on anterior viewing indicates that the pelvis is rotated anticlockwise, which corresponds with the patient's left ilium being closer to the examiner on posterior viewing (figure 7.8*c*).

When rotation occurs around the hip (coxal) joint, it is referenced according to whether it falls forward or backward in the transverse plane, and the terms *forward* and *backward* are always used to describe movement of the ilium opposite to the weight-bearing leg. Thus, when the left leg is the pivot point, to describe the pelvis of a patient

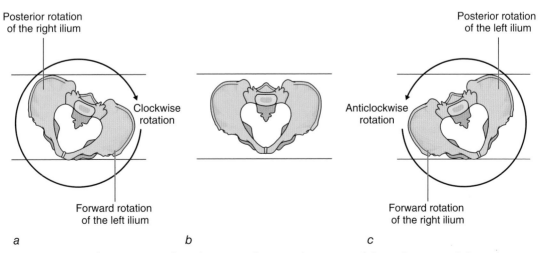

Figure 7.8 Pelvic rotation when the point of axis is the center of the pelvis, as in bilateral stance, with (*a*) clockwise rotation, (*b*) neutral position, and (*c*) anticlockwise rotation.

as having right forward rotation would mean the right ilium has pivoted anteriorly (figure 7.9a), whereas someone with right backward rotation displays posterior rotation of the right ilium (figure 7.9c) on the left leg. The degree of movement is greater than when it occurs in bilateral stance but is again exaggerated for the purposes of illustration here. Where the right leg is the pivot point, left forward rotation denotes that the left ilium is anterior (figure 7.10a) and left backward rotation denotes the left ilium is posterior (figure 7.10c).

Interestingly, observation that the client's right ilium is closer to you when viewing a client posteriorly (or the client's left ilium is closer to you when viewing the client anteriorly), for example, could be because the client is pivoting on the left leg and the pelvis is posteriorly rotated (figure 7.9c) or because the client is pivoting on the right leg and the pelvis is anteriorly rotated figure 7.10a). Observe from figures 7.9a and 7.10a that, irrespective of which leg is fixed, forward rotation of the pelvis corresponds with internal rotation of the femur of the supporting leg, and posterior rotation corresponds with external rotation of the femur (figures 7.9c and 7.10c). Prolonged internal rotation of the femur could result in shortening of the internal hip rotator muscles; prolonged external rotation of the femur could correspond with shortening of the external hip rotator muscles and may affect hip function.

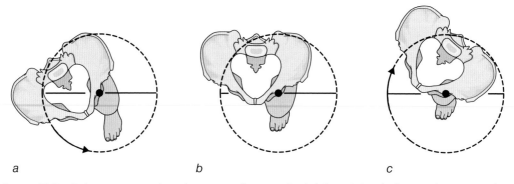

a   b   c

Figure 7.9 Pelvic rotation when the point of axis is the left leg: (a) right forward rotation, (b) neutral position and (c) right backward rotation.

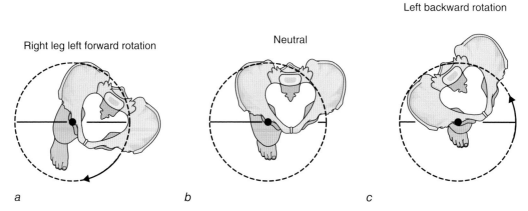

Right leg left forward rotation   Neutral   Left backward rotation

a   b   c

Figure 7.10 Pelvic rotation when the point of axis is the right leg: (a) left forward rotation, (b) neutral position and (c) left backward rotation.

Consequences of a Rotated Pelvis

Central to the body, rotation of the pelvis affects (and is affected by) the lower limbs and the torso. For the purposes of simplicity, consider what happens to the lower limbs when pelvic rotation occurs about a central point, as in figure 7.8b. When the pelvis is in a neutral position, forces are transmitted equally through the lower limbs and eventually through the feet (figure 7.11b). Clockwise rotation corresponds with increased supination of the right foot, inversion of the forefoot of the right foot and increased pressure on the lateral side of the foot; there is increased pronation of the left foot, although pressure through the lateral and medial sides of the left foot remains approximately equal (figure 7.11a). Rotation of the pelvis to anticlockwise corresponds with increased supination of the left foot and increased pressure on the lateral side of the left foot due to inversion of the forefoot; pressure through the right foot remains roughly equal, but there is increased pronation (figure 7.11c). Prolonged unequal pressure through the foot could adversely affect joints of the lower limb. For more information on postural change in the feet and ankles, see the sections on pes planus, pes cavus, pes valgus and pes varus in chapter 8.

The tibia is torsioned with pelvic rotation, albeit to a minor degree. You can demonstrate this for yourself when you stand with weight equally distributed through both feet and rotate your pelvis clockwise and then anticlockwise. Notice how your knees and ankles feel. For more information on tibial torsion please, see the section on tibial torsion in chapter 8.

Forward rotation of the pelvis in right-leg weight bearing (that is, anterior motion of the left ilium) produces compensatory lumbar spine rotation to the left; backward rotation produces lumbar spine rotation to the right. As the pelvis rotates clockwise,

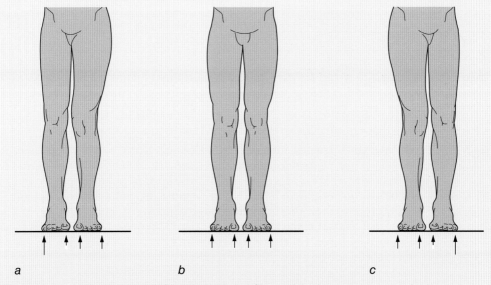

a   b   c

Figure 7.11 Change in pressure through the feet with pelvic rotation: *(a)* clockwise rotation, *(b)* neutral pelvis position (pressure through the feet is equal) and *(c)* anticlockwise rotation.

(continued)

Consequences of a Rotated Pelvis *(continued)*

the torso and shoulders follow suit. Again, you can demonstrate the effect of this for yourself in standing. Slowly turn your pelvis clockwise and observe how your shoulders rotate in a similar fashion. To face forward, the head and neck need to then rotate anticlockwise. So there is a kind of corkscrewing motion through the torso from pelvis to lumbar spine to thoracic spine to shoulders, neck and eventually head. You can see now why some therapists believe that to address postural asymmetry in other parts of the body it is always necessary to begin with the pelvis.

All of the muscles associated with each of these body parts are affected, some of which are presented in tables 7.3 and 7.4.

Table 7.3   Muscle Lengths Associated With Forward Rotated Pelvis in Right-Leg Weight Bearing

Area	Shortened muscles	Lengthened muscles
Trunk muscles	Right quadratus lumborum Right lumbar erector spinae Left thoracic erector spinae	Left quadratus lumborum Left lumbar erector spinae Right thoracic erector spinae
Hip muscles	Right hip medial rotators: anterior portion of gluteus medius, tensor fasciae latae Right hip adductors Possibly other muscles that contribute to medial rotation of the right hip: medial hamstrings, gluteus minimus, pectineus	Left hip lateral rotators: obturator internus, obturator externus, gemellus superior, gemellus inferior, piriformis, quadratus femoris, gluteus maximus

Table 7.4   Muscle Lengths Associated With Forward Rotated Pelvis in Left-Leg Weight Bearing

Area	Shortened muscles	Lengthened muscles
Trunk muscles	Left quadratus lumborum Left lumbar erector spinae Right thoracic erector spinae	Right quadratus lumborum Right lumbar erector spinae Left thoracic erector spinae
Hip muscles	Left hip medial rotators: anterior portion of gluteus medius, tensor fasciae latae Left hip adductors Possibly other muscles that contribute to medial rotation of the left hip: medial hamstrings, gluteus minimus, pectineus	Right hip lateral rotators: obturator internus, obturator externus, gemellus superior, gemellus inferior, piriformis, quadratus femoris, gluteus maximus

TIP As you learnt from the 'consequences' section, pelvic rotation produces a corkscrewing effect on the entire body. The result of this is that muscles throughout the body are affected and should be individually assessed for length. The greater the degree of rotation, the more muscles are likely to be affected, and to a greater degree.

What You Can Do as a Therapist

For the techniques described here, use tables 7.3 and 7.4 to help you decide whether the muscles you intend to treat are likely to be left-side or right-side muscles, and assess the length of these for yourself.

- Massage shortened tissues in an attempt to lengthen them. These are the trunk muscles (quadratus lumborum and the lumbar and thoracic erector spinae) and the following hip muscles: anterior portion of gluteus medius, tensor fasciae latae and hip adductors.

- Other muscles that might contribute to medial rotation of the hip are medial hamstrings, gluteus minimus and pectineus. Massage to quadratus lumborum and erector spinae unilaterally could be performed with the client in a side-lying position (figure 4.8b), and massage to thoracic or lumbar erector spinae unilaterally can be performed with the client seated (figure 4.6c). The advantage of using a seated position is that your client can flex or rotate away from you in such a way as to facilitate a stretch on these tissues as you massage. Massage to tensor fasciae latae (figure 8.2d), gluteus minimus and the anterior portion of gluteus medius could be performed with the client in a side-lying position, using static pressures to help lengthen these relatively smaller muscles.

- Passively stretch shortened muscles as previously, such as quadratus lumborum in supine (figure 8.2d) or side-lying positions (figure 4.8b), and the lumbar and thoracic erector spinae and the following hip muscles: anterior portion of gluteus medius, tensor fasciae latae and hip adductors.

- As you read in the section on consequences, you may wish to address tension in muscles superior or inferior to the pelvis if you have assessed these and found them to be shortened. For example, you could palpate and massage the oblique muscles (figure 4.8d).

- Explain to your client how he could use pelvic blocks to rest on as a corrective tool. Some therapists choose to massage clients whilst the client is resting on blocks, provided this is comfortable. Use of blocks in this way facilitates correction of the pelvis in addition to that provided by the massage of shortened tissues.

- Consider using MFR rocking technique, which is believed to help with pelvic realignment.

- Consider referring your client for gait analysis or to a podiatrist where you have identified lower-limb problems.

What Your Client Can Do

- Identify and avoid causal factors especially in prolonged sitting and standing where there is an element of spinal rotation, whether this is fixed or repetitive.

- Use pelvic blocks when resting. Known as padded wedges, pelvic wedges or pelvic blocks, these are simple pieces of firm foam that have been used for a chiropractic technique known as sacro-occipital technique. These are used to help overcome pelvic torsion (see the laterally raised pelvic posture in the next section) and either deliberately stress or de-stress the sacroiliac joint for the purposes of reducing pain. In chiropractic, two blocks are used to counter torsion and imbalances in the pelvis as the result of leg length discrepancy and are positioned in a specific manner. Use of blocks has been shown on X-ray to alter pelvic position (Klingensmith and Blum 2003). A single block could be useful in countering a rotated pelvis—that is, a pelvis rotated around the central spine axis—by facilitating a lengthening of shortened tissues whilst a client is relaxing with a block in place. Alternatively, a client could practice with a small, rolled-up towel or firm sponge, following the description provided here:

- If the pelvis is rotated clockwise (figure 7.12a), placing a block beneath the left ASIS in the prone position blocks clockwise rotation and repositions the pelvis into a more symmetrical position (figure 7.12b). If the pelvis is rotated anticlockwise (figure 7.12c), a block is needed beneath the right ASIS; again, this repositions the pelvis so that it is more neutral (figure 7.12d). Can you see how, if resting supine, a block would need to be positioned beneath the posterior of the right ilium in order to neutralize a clockwise-rotated pelvis (figure 7.12f) for this to become neutral, or beneath the left posterior ilium when treating anticlockwise rotation (figure 7.12g) to facilitate realignment (figure 7.12h)? Whether a patient rests prone or supine when using a block is a matter of personal preference.

- Actively stretch shortened muscles, such as quadratus lumborum and lumbar and thoracic erector spinae in supine (figure 4.9a) or seated (figure 4.9b) positions, and internal rotators of the hip on the weight-bearing-leg side.

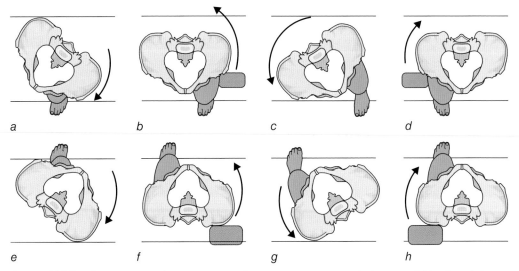

Figure 7.12 Correcting pelvic rotation in the prone position with the use of blocks : (a) Clockwise rotation brings the left iliac crest anterior; (b) placing a block under the left ASIS prevents further rotation and neutralizes the pelvis; (c) anticlockwise rotation brings the right iliac crest anterior; (d) a block under the right ASIS in the prone position prevents further rotation and neutralizes the pelvis. In the supine position (e) there is greater pressure on the posterior right ilium in clockwise rotation; (f) placing a block beneath the right posterior ilium neutralizes the pelvis; (g) there is greater pressure on the posterior left ilium in anticlockwise rotation; and (h) a block beneath the left posterior ilium neutralizes the pelvis.

Laterally Tilted Pelvis

In a laterally tilted pelvis the innominate bones (ilium, ischium and pubis) on one side of the pelvis are superior to those on the other side in the frontal plane. It is as if the pelvis has been hitched up on one side, and that is often what is most apparent when viewing a client posteriorly (figure 7.13a) or anteriorly (figure 7.13c). Right- and left-side anatomical landmarks are no longer horizontal (figure 7.13b).

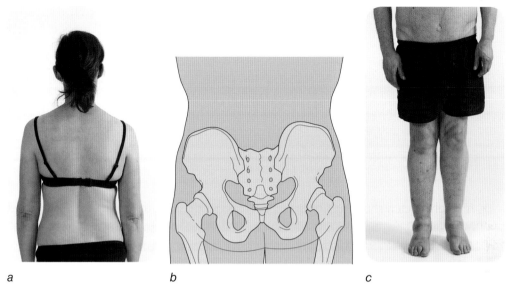

a   b   c

Figure 7.13 Laterally raised pelvis: (a) raised on the right, (b) anatomical landmarks are no longer horizontal, and (c) raised on the left.

Table 7.5   Muscle Lengths Associated With Laterally Tilted Pelvis Raised on the Right

Area	Shortened muscles	Lengthened muscles
Lumbar spine	Right quadratus lumborum Right erector spinae Right external oblique	Left quadratus lumborum Left erector spinae Left external oblique
Hip	Right hip adductors Left hip abductors	Left hip adductors Right hip abductors

TIP The iliotibial band and whole of the lateral side of the leg may be tight on the side of the pelvis that is lowered, corresponding with shortened hip abductors on that side.

What You Can Do as a Therapist

- Acknowledge that where pelvic asymmetry is the result of leg length discrepancy, therapeutic intervention may be limited.

- Help your client to identify factors that may be contributing to hip hitching. This could be an unleveled sitting surface at a workstation or improper lifting techniques (Klingensmith and Blum 2003). Even something as simple as sitting on a wallet that is too thick can contribute to pelvic imbalance (Viggiani et al. 2014).

- Help to lengthen shortened tissues using massage. There are many ways to do this including massage to quadratus lumborum in side lying (figure 4.8b) and massage to hip adductors (figure 7.14a). To help relax and lengthen hip abductors, static pressures are an option (figure 7.14b); this may be suitable for those clients who feel uncomfortable receiving gluteal massage.

Consequences of a Laterally Tilted Pelvis

Perhaps one of the most significant consequences of this posture is that it corresponds with torsion of the ilia. This phenomenon has been investigated by researchers interested in the consequences of leg length discrepancy, a common cause of a laterally tilted pelvis, especially where this coincides with back pain. In previous sections of this book, symmetrical movement of the pelvis has been assumed where there is anterior pelvic tilt (See Anterior Pelvic Tilt at the start of this chapter) or posterior pelvic tilt (See Posterior Pelvic Tilt earlier in this chapter) in the sagittal plane, where the innominates move either anteriorly or posteriorly, respectively. However, it is possible for innominates to move and be fixed unilaterally and in opposite directions. In this kind of torsion, the innominate moves posteriorly on the side of the long leg (raised side of the pelvis) and anteriorly on the side of the short leg (lower side of the pelvis) (Cooperstein and Lew 2009). One way to think of this movement is akin to the Rubik's Cube toy, where opposite sides of the cub are rotated simultaneously in opposite directions. In previous sections we have seen that when the sacrum moves with respect to the ilia. This is known as nutation and counternutation (see figure 7.4). Pelvic torsion also occurs at the sacroiliac joint but describes movement of the ilia moving with respect to the sacrum where left and right ilia move in opposite directions in the sagittal plane. Pelvic torsion resulting from leg length discrepancy creates asymmetry in lumbosacral facet joints, wedging of the fifth lumbar vertebra, concavities in vertebral body end plates, and scoliosis (Klingensmith and Blum 2003). Such torsion is associated with back pain but it is not clear why this is so. Dysfunction in the sacroiliac joints is associated with back pain (Cohen 2005). Correlations have been found between pelvic torsion and the position of the lower jaw (Lippold et al. 2007). This has implications for the treatment of patients with orthodontic conditions such as malocclusion.

- Passively stretch shortened tissues. For example, to stretch quadratus lumborum you could use supine (figure 4.8a) or side-lying (figure 4.8b) positions and instruct your client to drop the hip, thus stretching quadratus lumborum on that side. It helps if you demonstrate and have your client practice dropping the hip before you attempt the stretch. There are many ways to stretch hip adductors unilaterally and could involve knee flexion or extension (figure 7.14c).

- Consider myofascial release, deep tissue massage or passive stretching to the iliotibial band on the side of the pelvis that is lower, corresponding with shortness in gluteals on that side.

- Teach your client the active stretches and simple exercises illustrated in What Your Client Can Do.

- Consider referral to a podiatrist if you suspect leg length discrepancy is a contributing factor.

What Your Client Can Do
- Identify causal factors (e.g., sitting with legs crossed, sitting with the torso slightly rotated, leaning backwards, leaning to one side, carrying a heavy bag on one side).

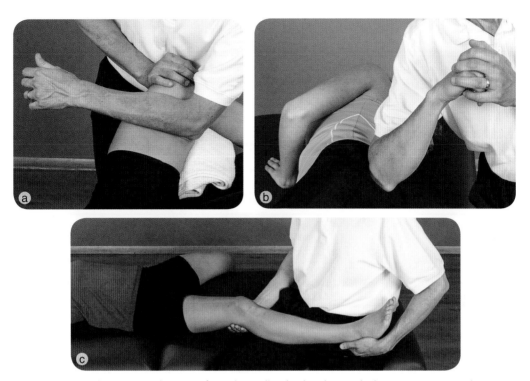

Figure 7.14 Therapist techniques for a laterally tilted pelvis include (a) massage to hip adductors, (b) static pressure to hip abductors, and (c) unilateral passive hip adductor stretches with the knee extended.

Each of these shortens the quadratus lumborum, a prime lateral flexor of the spine and a hip hitcher.

- Practice dropping the hip, lowering the side that is usually raised. This can be practiced in the supine position (figure 7.15a). Clients often benefit from instruction with this exercise. For example, encourage a client to try to touch an imaginary object that is just out of reach of his foot on the side of the pelvis that is raised. In this example, the patient is stretching down with his left leg because his left ilium is raised.

- Using active stretches, lengthen the quadratus lumborum and lumbar erector spinae on the side on which the pelvis is raised. There are many ways to do this. For example, simply reaching the arm up whilst sitting (figure 7.15b) elevates the lower rib to which the quadratus lumborum is attached. Sometimes when clients practice supine stretches such as in figures 4.8b and 4.9, they become aware of their pelvic asymmetry when they discover it is easier to stretch to one side than to the other.

- Using active adductor stretches, lengthen adductors on the side on which the pelvis is raised.

- Use a therapy ball to apply static pressure to self-trigger tender points in hip abductors on the side on which the pelvis is lower (figure 7.15c). Note that for many clients, resting on a tennis ball as shown is painful, and some clients cannot get into this position. An alternative is to suggest that your client simply place the trigger ball or tennis ball against a wall and do the exercise whilst standing.

- Use a foam roller and actively stretch the iliotibial band (see figure 7.15d) on the side of the pelvis that is lower, corresponding with shortness in gluteals on that side.
- Where pelvic torsion has been identified, use blocks as described in the section on rotated pelvic posture (see figure 7.12).

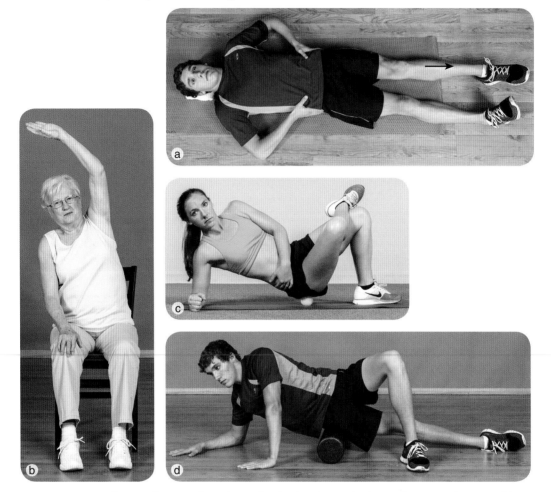

Figure 7.15 Client techniques for a laterally tilted pelvis include (a) dropping the raised hip to stretch quadratus lumborum, (b) stretching quadratus lumborum and lumbar erector spinae muscles in a seated position, (c) using a tennis ball to deactivate trigger of gluteals and (d) using a foam roller on the gluteals.

Closing Remarks

In this chapter you learnt about four common pelvic postures: anterior tilted pelvis, posteriorly tilted pelvis, rotated pelvis and laterally raised pelvis. The anatomical features of each appear along with photographic examples and illustrations. The consequences of each posture are described, and you learnt that the position of the pelvis plays a significant role in the posture of the lower limbs and torso. For each pathology, a table presents lists of shortened and lengthened muscles that can help you plan your treatments.

Lower Limb

The 10 postures covered in this chapter are internal rotation of hip, genu recurvatum (knee hyperextension), genu flexum (knee flexion), genu varum (bow legs), genu valgum (knock knees), tibial torsion, flatfoot (pes planus), high arches in feet (pes caves), pronation in feet (pes valgus) and supination in feet (pes varus).

Internal Rotation of the Hip

Internal rotation of the hip is internal rotation around the long axis of the femur. A patient with this posture may have a characteristic toe-in foot position, where the tibia is also internally rotated, or the foot position may be neutral. Whether the foot position is toe-in or neutral, the patella faces inward, which is one way to identify this posture. However, unlike some of the other postures with signs that are visibly apparent, the degree of inward rotation of the femur is more difficult to identify from postural assessment alone, and for this reason muscle length tests are important for determining whether a patient has a reduction in external hip rotation, which is a corresponding finding with this posture.

It is important to note that internal rotation of the hip is not the same as internal torsion of the femur. Femoral torsion is rotation *within* a bone itself, a twisting of the bone, whereas internal rotation of the hip occurs between bones, at the coxofemoral joint. Each results in a change in the orientation of the femoral condyles in the transverse plane. So observing the client's knees anteriorly and posteriorly can be helpful in identifying internal rotation of the hip. With both internal rotation of the hip and internal femoral torsion, the lateral femoral condyle is orientated more anteriorly than normal and the medial femoral condyle is orientated more posteriorly. In this patient (figure 8.1a), the lateral femoral condyle of the left femur is anteriorly orientated and disappears from a posterior view, whereas the medial femoral condyle is posteriorly orientated and appears more prominent. This indicates internal rotation of the left hip or internal femoral torsion on that side.

To help you identify internal rotation when viewing a client posteriorly, imagine the popliteal spaces as if they were the headlights on a car (figure 8.1b). Kneeling squarely

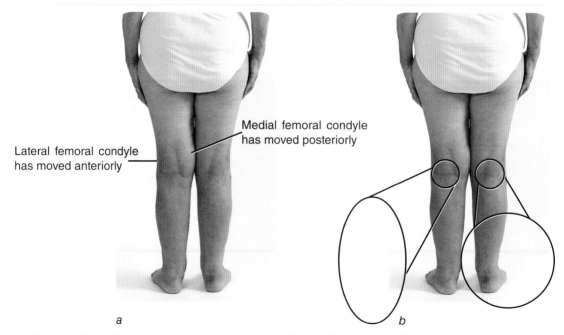

Medial femoral condyle has moved posteriorly

Lateral femoral condyle has moved anteriorly

a

b

Figure 8.1 *(a)* A patient with internal rotation of the left hip (internal femoral torsion); *(b)* imagining the popliteal spaces as vehicle headlights.

behind your client, but about 2 meters from them, ask yourself where the headlight beams would fall. Would a beam be directed towards you (indicating normal tibio-femoral alignment) or to one side (indicating hip rotation, or femoral torsion)? Observe that the popliteal spaces on this patient's right and left knees are not orientated in the same direction; a beam from the left-knee headlight would fall to your left, whereas the beam from the right-knee headlight would fall closer to you.

It is tempting to conclude that a person standing with forward-facing feet does not have any internal rotation at the hip joint. Remember that in normal standing, the feet turn outwards slightly by about 6 to 8 degrees, so a patient with feet facing forwards

Consequences of Internal Rotation of the Hip

With increased internal hip rotation there is corresponding decreased external rotation in the coxofemoral joint. Internal rotators are shortened and external rotators are lengthened. Both muscle groups may be weakened because they are not functioning at their optimal length or within their optimal range. Weakness in external rotators of the hip is associated with musculoskeletal disorders of the knee such as patellofemoral joint pain syndrome and noncontact injury to the anterior cruciate ligament in adolescent girls (Neumann 2010). Imbalance in muscles around the hip joint could affect function of the joint and ultimately affect not only gait but also functional and sporting activities.

Femoral torsion can be a contributing factor to internal rotation of the hip. The degree of femoral torsion is described as an angle that is formed by a line drawn longitudinally through the neck of the femur superimposed over a line drawn between the femoral condyles. This angle is usually 10 to 15 degrees but varies widely. An increase in torsion angle is called anteversion. Anteversion can cause compensatory change in the hip joint and affect weight bearing, muscle biomechanics and hip joint stability and may also create dysfunction at the knee and foot (Levangie and Norkin 2001).

Internal rotation of the hip changes the normal orientation of the femoral head within the acetabulum. Prolonged alteration in the distribution of forces through the articular surfaces of the hip joint could predispose the joint to degenerative changes in the bone, articular cartilage and connective tissue. Internal rotation of the hip threatens to pinch anterior hip structures, causing pain.

With internal rotation of the femur there is abnormal orientation of the knee joint. This is exacerbated where there is a neutral foot position because this requires external rotation of the tibia in cases where internal rotation of the femur is present. Altered hip and knee biomechanics alter both walking and running ability and could therefore adversely affect participation in recreational and sporting activities. Where internal rotation is due to torsional deformity of the femur, this could contribute to arthritis in the knee joint: Internal femoral torsion increases pressure on the lateral facet, producing anterior knee pain and patellofemoral arthritis. There may be lateral patellar subluxation.

Internal rotation of the hip is often accompanied by subtalar pronation of the foot, and this too causes problems (see later in this chapter for more information).

could have an internally rotated hip or internal tibial torsion, or both. (A section on tibial torsion appears later in this chapter.)

The subject of internal hip rotation can be confusing because both internal rotation of the femur and internal femoral torsion contribute to torsion of the entire lower limb. Inward rotation of the entire lower limb may be the result of a combination of factors at the coxofemoral and knee joints and within the femur and tibia. As with many of the postures described in this book, it is important to clarify the degree of internal rotation you suspect using muscle length tests rather than to rely on postural assessment alone.

Table 8.1 Muscle Lengths Associated With Internal Rotation of the Hip

Area	Shortened muscles	Lengthened muscles
Hip	Tensor fasciae latae	Gluteus maximus
	Gluteus minimus	Gluteus medius (posterior fibers)
	Gluteus medius (anterior fibers)	Piriformis
	Adductor longus	Quadratus femoris
	Adductor brevis	Obturator
	Adductor magnus	Gemelli muscles
	Pectineus	Psoas
	Gracilis	Sartorius

TIP Note that piriformis, posterior fibers of gluteus minimus and anterior fibers of gluteus maximus change from being external to internal rotators as the hip is progressively flexed.

What You Can Do as a Therapist

- Acknowledge that where internal rotation is the result of bony anatomy, such as femoral torsion, non-surgical intervention to correct internal hip rotation is limited.

- Apply passive stretches to internal rotators. Measured with the hip in flexion, normal internal rotation of the hip is 30 to 40 degrees and external rotation is 40 to 60 degrees (Magee 2002). The supine (figure 8.2a) and prone (figure 8.2b) positions commonly used to assess for the degree of hip rotation can also be used to apply passive stretches. When performing passive stretches in either position, you will need to move your client's leg as if testing for external rotation. Arrows on each diagram indicate the direction you move the leg to facilitate the stretch. Where there is short-ness in internal rotator muscles, the degree to which you will be able to rotate the leg into external rotation will be reduced. Gentle overpressure can be applied at this point to stretch the internal rotator muscles. Note that there is considerable differ-ence in reported findings for measurements of hip range of motion (Kouyoumdjian et al. 2012), so take care not to overstretch a client's tissues in an attempt to reach a norm value. Figure 8.2c shows a good way to hold the leg when attempting to stretch internal rotators in the supine position. Observe that the therapist is taking care not to invert the client's foot with his left hand and has adopted a stance that facilitates leverage. This position may not be appropriate for all of your clients, but when it is used, it is more stable when performed on the floor than on a treatment couch.

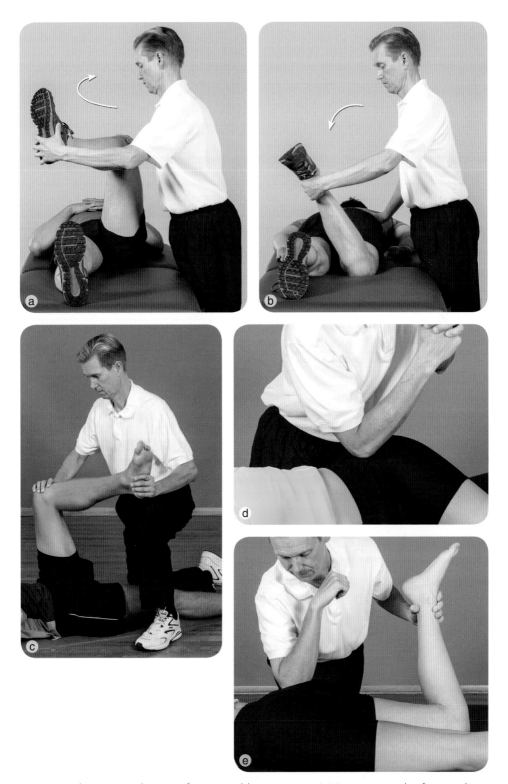

Figure 8.2 Therapist techniques for internal hip rotation: *(a)* Passive stretch of internal rotators using supine and *(b)* prone positions require avoiding overstretching the lateral ankle ligaments when *(c)* performing this with the client supine. *(d)* Static pressure to tensor fasciae latae and *(e)* soft tissue release applied to gluteus medius can help lengthen these muscles.

- Stretching tensor fasciae latae may be particularly important in the treatment of internal hip rotation (Kendall et al. 1993). Static pressure to this small muscle (figure 8.2*d*) is one way to facilitate a reduction in tension in the muscle.

- Use soft tissue release to lengthen gluteus medius. With the hip in a neutral position, gently lock the muscle using your thumb or elbow (figure 8.2e) and then use your other hand to move your client's leg (as if testing for external rotation) whilst maintaining the lock.

- Massage and passively stretch adductors on the affected side. (For examples, please see figure 7.14.)

- Address trigger points in gluteals and adductor muscles where you find these.

- Use MFR longitudinal leg pulls because these can relax all muscles of the hip joint and the entire lower limb before using some of the previously described techniques.

- Consider referring your client to a fitness instructor for supervision of exercises to strengthen external hip rotators.

- Consider experimenting with a device such as the SERF strap (stability through external rotation of the femur). Exercise caution when using such straps because these alter the alignment of not only the hip but also the knee, ankle and foot, which may have negative as well as positive consequences. It is essential for clients using a SERF strap to also perform exercises to strengthen external hip rotators on a regular basis.

- Consider referral to a podiatrist because orthotics may be helpful in correcting the degree of rotation.

What Your Client Can Do

- Identify and avoid postures that contribute to internal hip rotation. For example, avoid standing pigeon-toed, twisting the feet around chair legs (figure 8.3*a*), sleeping in the prone position where there is a tendency to turn the lower limb inwards, or sitting in the W position, a childhood posture believed by many to contribute to the development of internal rotation of the hip.

- Actively stretch internal rotators of the hip using stretches such as in figure 8.3*b*. Where internal rotators are particularly tight, it can be difficult to lower the affected thigh to a horizontal position. Gentle pressure may be applied to the knee, increasing the stretch of muscles such as piriformis and hip adductors.

- Actively stretch tensor fasciae latae. Standing stretches are often prescribed to clients wishing to stretch this muscle and the ITB. However, these are not always effective. Using a tennis ball to self-trigger this small muscle may help to relax and lengthen it.

- Actively stretch hip adductor muscles. Some clients might feel a stretch when performing the gluteal stretch simply because the hip is abducted in this position.

- Strengthen external rotators of the hip using exercises such as prone hip extension and bridging. Note that many exercises strengthen external hip rotators, and it may be helpful to work with a fitness instructor or other qualified person to ensure that the exercises are being performed correctly. This may be particularly important where internal rotation is unilateral. Patients with recent lumbar herniation should not perform prone hip extension.

- Consider swimming using the breaststroke. This stroke requires external rotation of the femur and could assist in strengthening lateral rotators and possibly encourage a lengthening of internal rotators.

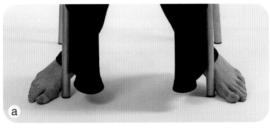

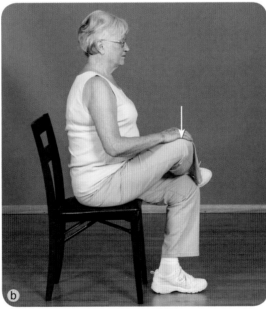

Figure 8.3 Client techniques for internal rotation of the hip include avoidance of posture likely to contribute to internal rotation such as *(a)* sitting with the feet wrapped around chair legs and *(b)* stretches to the internal rotators of the hip and hip adductor muscles.

Genu Recurvatum

Commonly termed *knee hyperextension*, this posture describes extension at the knee (tibiofemoral) joint greater than neutral or zero degrees when weight bearing. Viewed laterally, an imaginary line drawn vertically from just anterior to the lateral malleolus bisects the fibula longitudinally in normal knee posture (figure 8.4a). In the genu recurvatum posture a larger portion of the calf falls posterior to this line, which no longer bisects the leg (figure 8.4b). Observe from this patient with mild genu recurvatum (figure 8.4c) that increased plantar flexion (decreased dorsiflexion) at the ankle is a common finding.

This posture is best identified by viewing your client in the sagittal plane. Also, observation of a prominent calf and popliteal space when you view your client posteriorly, and a downward pointing patella that appears compressed when you view your client anteriorly, are additional hints. This posture is associated with excessive femoral internal rotation, genu varum or genu valgum, tibial varum and excessive subtalar joint pronation, all more apparent when you view your client anteriorly.

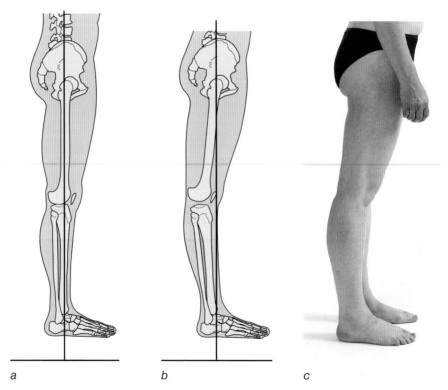

a b c

Figure 8.4 Genu recurvatum posture: *(a)* normal knee alignment, *(b)* knee alignment in genu recurvatum and *(c)* mild genu recurvatum.

Consequences of Genu Recurvatum

In this posture there is tension in posterior knee structures (such as popliteus) and compression of anterior structures (such as the patellofemoral joint). As a consequence, adults who stand in knee hyperextension may have pain in the popliteal space (Kendall et al. 1993) and patellofemoral pain. People with hypermobility have laxity in knee ligaments and stand in the genu recurvatum posture. The knee is the most painful joint in people with knee hypermobility, and patellofemoral pain syndrome is a common problem (Tinkle 2008).

Additionally, the normal kinematics of the knee are affected by alteration of tibiofemoral mechanics. In normal weight bearing, the femur rolls anteriorly and glides posteriorly on the fixed tibia, but in knee hyperextension the femur tilts forward, resulting in anterior compression of the femur and tibia. In weight bearing, capsular and ligamentous structures of the posterior knee are at risk of injury, and this in turn may lead to functional gait deficits. Patients with genu recurvatum posture walk more slowly than normal and many have higher knee extensor torque values than those with normal knee posture (Kerrigan et al. 1996).

Other joints are also affected. There is increased hip extension and decreased ankle dorsiflexion, both of which are likely to affect gait and impair sporting performance that relies on lower-limb agility. At the hip there can be excessive anterior tilt. This posture results in gait deviation and requires greater effort to maintain forward momentum (Fish and Kosta 1998).

The quadriceps and soleus muscles are shortened and knee flexor muscles are lengthened. Imbalance between knee flexors and extensors compromises the function and stability of both the knee and hip joints. Stretching of popliteus reduces its ability to rotate the leg medially on the thigh and flex the knee and therefore affects optimal knee function. There may be proprioceptive deficit near the end of range of extension (Loudon 1998). Patients may feel the sensation of knee instability.

A positive correlation between genu recurvatum and anterior cruciate ligament injury in female athletes has been found (Loudon 1998). Genu recurvatum posture may predispose female athletes to overuse injuries of the knee (Devan et al. 2004). Knee hyperextension may be prevalent in some swimmers, and it has been postulated that this is the result of overstretching of the cruciate ligaments due to repetitive kicking. This posture gives a greater range of anterior-to-posterior motion at the knee, but it is not clear whether genu recurvatum is advantageous to swimmers (Bloomfield et al. 1994).

Table 8.2 Muscle Lengths Associated With Hyperextended Knee Posture

Area	Shortened muscles	Lengthened muscles
Thigh	Quadriceps	Semitendinosus Semimembranosus Biceps femoris
Leg	Soleus	Popliteus Gastrocnemius

What You Can Do as a Therapist

- Instruct your client in good postural alignment, helping her to identify those times when she stands with the knees locked out in the hyperextended posture.

- Apply tape to the posterior knee. Rather than prevent hyperextension, the purpose of taping is to provide sensory feedback in order to help your client identify when she has a tendency to hyperextend. This may be particularly useful when treating dancers with hypermobility syndrome (Knight 2011). Ultimately, self-correction of the posture is preferable to reliance on tape, which should be used only in the short term whilst your client is learning to avoid hyperextension. Tape can be applied in a variety of ways, such as a single wide strip (figure 8.5a), two narrower strips (figure 8.5b) or a cross (figure 8.5c). Whichever method you choose, apply the tape with the knee in a neutral position. Rather than attempt this with your client standing, ask her to lie face down, where the knee usually rests in a neutral position.

- Passively stretch quadriceps. There are many ways to do this, such as in the prone position, which stabilizes the pelvis to prevent anterior tilt and lumbar extension, which otherwise reduces the effectiveness of the stretch and can be uncomfortable (figure 7.7b).

- Apply deep tissue massage to relax and lengthen quadriceps.

- If you think it falls within your professional remit, provide exercises to strengthen knee flexors. These could include regular hamstring and calf strengthening or asking your client to perform small amounts of knee flexion against the gentle resistance of your hands placed just beneath the knee (figure 8.5d) within a small range of motion.

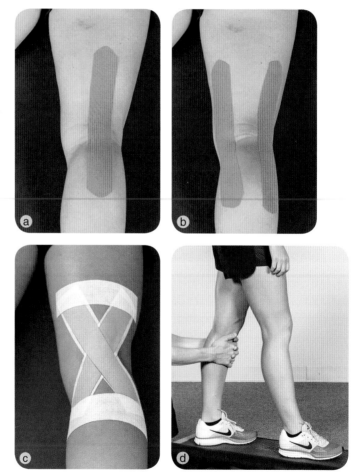

Figure 8.5 Therapist techniques for genu recurvatum include taping using (a) single, (b) double or (c) cross-shaped applications and (d) knee strengthening exercises.

Take care of your own posture when facilitating this exercise, perhaps by asking your client to stand on a raised platform so that you do not have to stoop so much.

- Consider referral to a physiotherapist for proprioceptive training and gait training.

- Consider referral to a podiatrist who may have suggestions for treatment to limit the extent of hyperextension during daily activities. For example, using a small elevated heel creates knee flexion during walking, which slows gait but can be helpful in preventing hyperextension. Use of orthotics under the medial border of the foot can help limit subtalar pronation, a posture associated with genu recurvatum. AFOs, rigid ankle and foot boots, are sometimes prescribed to help correct genu recurvatum whilst walking; although these reduce the energy requirement of walking, they do not always reduce extensor movement at the knee (Kerrigan et al. 1996).

- Consider referral to a sport therapist for sport-specific drills to help your client master a flexed knee position during fast, dynamic movements.

What Your Client Can Do

- Become conscious of knee postures during everyday activities.

- Practice good knee alignment in static postures. For example, take particular care with standing postures by avoiding locking out the knee; avoid placing the ankles on a footstool when seated because this allows the knee to sag into extension, stretching posterior tissues.

- Practice good knee alignment during dynamic functions such as standing up from a sitting position and stair climbing.

- To improve proprioception, practice single-leg balancing with the knee in proper alignment.

- Perform exercises to improve the strength ratio between knee flexors and extensors. Whilst balance between quadriceps and hamstrings may be crucial to the prevention of knee injury, unfortunately it is difficult to state the ideal strength ratio between these muscle groups because it depends not only on the sport but also on the angle of other joints (Alter 2004).

- Consider protecting the knees against hyperextension during sporting activities, especially those involving impact such as jumping.

- Avoid exercises and stretches that force the knee into extension. For example, take care with standing hamstring and calf stretches.

- Discuss which forms of sporting activity may be most suitable to someone with genu recurvatum posture. Prevention of knee hyperextension requires focused control of the joint and could be aggravated by sports involving fast movements. This posture may be disadvantageous to participation in field sports such as rugby, football, hockey and lacrosse (Bloomfield et al. 1994). It is likely to be disadvantageous for participation in jumping sports and sports that involve excessive loading of the lower limb. Clients with hyperextended knees would be better suited to activities such as tai chi, where movements are slow and controlled, rather than high-impact sports involving frequent changes of direction, such as racquet sports. Simple balancing exercises are beneficial to these clients because they adopt the neutral knee position and attempt to maintain it.

Genu Flexum

As the name indicates, in the genu flexum (flexed knee) posture a person bears weight through a knee that is flexed to a greater degree than is normal when standing. Less common than genu recurvatum, it is a posture observed in the elderly or in patients who have been sedentary and their knees have been allowed to rest in a flexed position for prolonged periods. Viewed laterally, an imaginary line drawn vertically from just anterior to the lateral malleolus bisects the tibia longitudinally in normal knee posture (figure 8.6a). In the genu flexum posture the knee itself falls anterior to this line, which no longer bisects the leg (figure 8.6b). This posture is best identified by viewing your client in the sagittal plane, as with the patient in figure 8.6c. Note the increased ankle dorsiflexion commonly associated with this posture.

What You Can Do as a Therapist

Caution is needed when attempting to address genu flexum after knee surgery and when working with clients who use wheelchairs or spend much of their time in a chair, such as someone who might be frail or recovering from illness or injury. For each of the techniques suggested, consider whether deep pressure (as might be used when applying soft tissue release or addressing trigger points) is contraindicated for your client; ensure that your client has sufficient balance when performing any standing exercises.

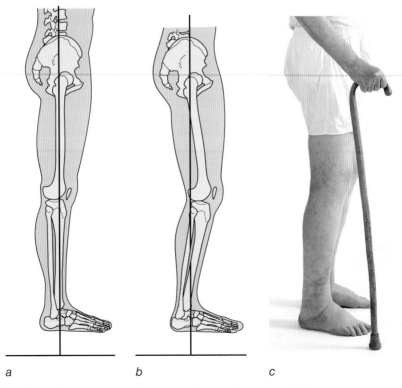

a　　　　　*b*　　　　　*c*

Figure 8.6　Genu flexum posture: *(a)* normal knee alignment, *(b)* knee alignment in genu flexum, and *(c)* genu flexum of the right leg.

Consequences of Genu Flexum

When the knee is extended, the collateral ligaments are relatively taut, helping to stabilize the joint. They slacken when the knee flexes and permit some axial rotation. Repeated weight bearing through a flexed knee could increase the likelihood of rotational injury to the knee.

Constant muscular effort is required for standing in knee flexion, which can be fatiguing. Constant contraction of the quadriceps has another disadvantage. This muscle exerts a pull on the tibia at the insertion of the tibial tuberosity, and this could lead to tenderness, or the development of unwanted teno-osseous pathology. There is increased pressure on the anterior aspect of the ankle due to increased dorsiflexion.

Prolonged unilateral knee flexion is associated with pronation of the foot and medial rotation of the contralateral thigh, plus ipsilateral hip drop (contralateral hip hitch), convexing of the spine toward the affected side, and contralateral drop of the shoulder (Kendall et al. 1993). For example, a patient with right knee flexion is more likely to have pronation of the left foot, internal rotation of the left thigh, a dropped hip on the right side but a raised hip on the left side and a dropped left shoulder.

Table 8.3   Muscle Lengths Associated With Genu Flexum Knee Posture

Area	Shortened muscles	Lengthened muscles
Thigh	Semitendinosus Semimembranosus Biceps femoris	Quadriceps
Leg	Popliteus	Soleus

- Recognize that intervention may be limited for clients where genu flexum results from abnormal high tone (e.g., spasticity associated with cerebral palsy).

- Passively release posterior knee tissues using myofascial release technique. This is an ideal technique to use for this posture where tissues on the back of the knee are tensed and pressure into the back of the knee must be avoided because of the presence of the popliteal artery and lymph nodes. A simple cross-hand technique could work well here, with one hand placed superior to the knee and one inferior to it.

- Passively stretch shortened muscles, in this case hamstrings and soleus. There are many ways to do this, including simple stretches held at the end of the existing range (figure 8.7). One of the advantages of this simple supine hamstring stretch is that it can be performed with the knee flexed and, instead of passively flexing the hip at the end of range, ask your client to extend the knee. Contraction of quadriceps will facilitate relaxation of the hamstrings, increasing knee extension without the need for further hip flexion.

- Apply massage to encourage a relaxation and lengthening of hamstrings and soleus. This could be deep tissue massage or soft tissue release to address tension you discover localized in specific tissues. Soft tissue release is useful here because

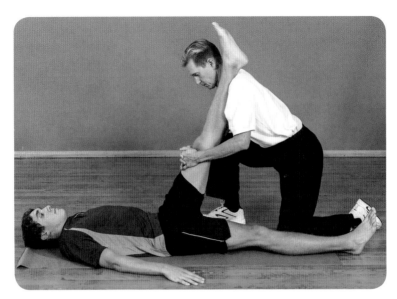

Figure 8.7 Therapist techniques for genu flexum include passive stretch of knee flexors.

it permits you to work within a range of knee flexion postures, stretching localized tissues only as far as is comfortable for your client.

- Treat any trigger points that you find in posterior tissues using localized static pressure and taking care not to press directly into the popliteal space.

- Genu flexum may be secondary to hip flexion (anterior tilt of the pelvis). If your assessments indicate an anteriorly tilted pelvis and shortened hip flexors, treat accordingly using the ideas put forward in chapter 7.

- Using the ideas set out in other sections of this book, treat the altered postures in other joints associated with genu flexum such as foot pronation, medial rotation of the hip, hip hitch and convexity of the spine.

What Your Client Can Do

- Rest in positions likely to stretch the posterior knee tissues. For example, using a footrest, the posterior knee is stretched through gravity (figure 8.8a). It is in the prone position, feet off the couch, and a light weight can be added to the ankle. Take care when using the prone position so as not to injure the front of the knee against the side of the couch or bed. This position is not suitable for clients with patellofemoral conditions when compression of the patella could be aggravating.

- Practice standing knee extension exercises using a stretchy band. Take care that the band is not too narrow because this could press into the back of the knee and cause pain. Active contraction of knee extensors in this manner encourages relaxation in the opposing muscle group, the knee flexors.

- Practice knee extension in supine (figure 8.8b). This is a good starting point for clients with pain or balance issues, for whom the previous exercise may be too demanding. Simply rest comfortably and attempt to press the back of the knee into the bed, floor or treatment couch. Some people place a bolster or small rolled-up towel beneath the ankle to provide leverage.

- Actively stretch the soleus muscle.

- Avoid prolonged sitting where possible unless it is with the legs outstretched and knees extended. If in a seated job, take short breaks and stand every hour to stretch the back of the leg.

- Active soft tissue release can be useful in addressing specific regions of tension in posterior thigh tissues; it is a technique that enables the client to self-treat the knee in flexion.

- Temporarily avoid sports that might perpetuate a flexed knee posture, such as rowing and cycling.

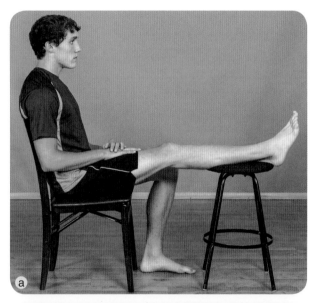

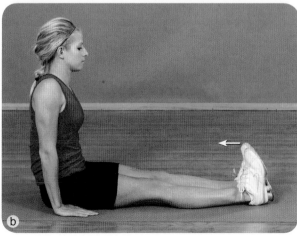

Figure 8.8 Client techniques for genu flexum include letting gravity stretch the posterior tissues in (a) sitting or (b) active knee extension in a supine position.

Genu Varum

The normal angle formed between the anatomical axis of the femur and the anatomical axis of the tibia on the medial side of the knee is approximately 195 degrees (Levangie and Norkin 2001). Popularly termed *bow legs*, genu varum is misalignment of the knee joint such that the medial tibiofemoral angle is *less than* 180 degrees. The severity of this posture can be determined by observing the distance between the medial femoral condyles when your client stands with the medial malleoli touching (figure 8.9*b*). Varum deformity can occur unilaterally also. Although the patient in figure 8.9*c* is not standing with the ankles touching, you can still see that the client has mild genu varum and slight bowing of the right tibia. Postural bow legs occur as the result of medial rotation of the femur and pronation of the foot (Kendall et al. 1993). In postural bow legs there is medial rotation of the hip joint, knee hyperextension and foot pronation.

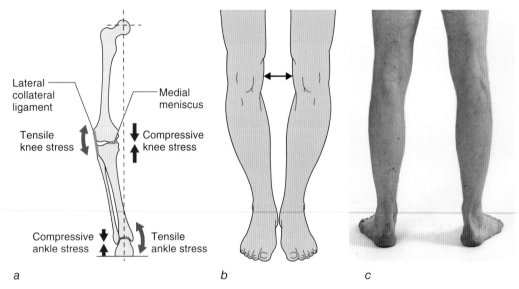

a *b* *c*

Figure 8.9 Genu varum: *(a)* gapping and compressive forces, *(b)* patient standing with medial malleoli touching, *(c)* mild genu varum and bowing of the right tibia.

Consequences of Genu Varum

In the genu varum posture there is increased tensile stress in the lateral side of the knee and medial side of the ankle and increased compressive forces on the medial side of the knee and lateral side of the ankle (figure 8.9*a*).

A way to appreciate the consequences of these strains is to imagine the gapping motion that has occurred in the lateral side of the joint (figure 8.9*a*). Gapping means that the lateral collateral ligament is tensed and possibly weakened, providing less stability and increasing the likelihood of lateral collateral ligament injury. The medial meniscus is compressed, possibly causing damage here too.

Being vertical, the mechanical axis of the knee means that during normal bilateral weight bearing, forces are transmitted through the centre of the knee joint distributed equally through the medial and lateral compartments. Misalignment of the joint shifts the transition of force to the medial aspect of the knee, which affects balance and gait and may predispose a patient to knee pathology. For example, some studies have found that knee malalignment is associated with higher rates of knee osteoarthritis (McWilliams et al. 2010). Whether a joint progresses to severe osteoarthritis depends on its existing state of vulnerability: A joint with mild osteoarthritis, for example, may be less vulnerable to the biomechanical effects of malalignment than a more damaged joint (Cerejo et al. 2002). If you imagine the mechanical axis of figure 8.9a as a bowstring, you can see how this posture gets its name and how it has a tendency to worsen in the genu varum posture.

As you can see from table 8.4, in the genu varum posture certain muscles are lengthened and others are shortened. Taking the posterior thigh alone, you can see that the iliotibial band is tensioned and lengthened compared to a normal posture, as is biceps femoris, whereas gracilis and semitendinosus are shortened. This may have little impact on day-to-day activities but could compromise a patient's participation in sport.

Additionally, not only are quadriceps shortened, but the genu varum posture also affects the direction of pull by the quadriceps on the patella. There may be a tendency for the patella to be pulled medially. Important for overall knee stability, altering the direction of pull of the patella could disrupt this bone's normal gliding mechanism and could lead to instability in the knee. In extreme cases the genu varum posture could contribute to degenerative changes in the patellofemoral joint.

The abnormal joint position is also likely to affect the normal glide and roll of the femur on the tibia that occurs during flexion and extension movements of the knee. During weight bearing there may be medial rotation in the leg and, in turn, the medial side of the foot can be elevated from the floor unless compensatory subtalar joint pronation occurs. Other compensatory movements may include eversion of the talus and pronation of the intertarsal joints as a means of regaining contact with the ground surface. This posture adversely affects balance and is significant especially in the elderly population in which genu varum is more common, as are falls. Genu varum deformity has been shown to increase normal postural sway in the mediolateral direction and increase risk of falls (Samaei et al. 2012).

Table 8.4   Muscle Lengths Associated With Genus Varum Knee Posture

Area	Shortened muscles	Lengthened muscles
Thigh	Quadriceps Internal hip rotators Gracilis Semitendinosus and semimembranosus relative to biceps femoris	Lateral rotators of the hip Biceps femoris relative to semitendinosus and semimembranosus
Leg	Fibulari (peroneal) muscles	Popliteus Tibialis posterior Long toe flexors

TIP The iliotibial band may be lengthened.

What You Can Do as a Therapist

■ Recognize that where bony change has occurred, such as bowing of the femur or tibia or both, non-surgical intervention is limited.

■ Where bow-leggedness appears to be postural only, with little or no anatomical change, encourage your client to identify and avoid those times when he may aggravate this posture (e.g., when shifting weight to the affected leg and permitting the knee to bow outwards).

■ Consider referring your client to a podiatrist, who may be able to offer specialist advice. For example, angled insoles can be used to transfer the load from the medial to the lateral compartment of the knee and perhaps alter the tibiofemoral angle. Lateral forefoot and rearfoot wedge insoles have been used to facilitate foot pronation (Gross 1995).

■ Consider referral to an exercise professional to assist with exercises to strengthen external rotators of the hip.

■ Although controversial, anecdotal evidence suggests that taping may be helpful in training gluteal muscles. The method shown here is based on that recommended by Langendoen and Sertel (2011). One at a time, apply two strips of tape from the proximal anterior thigh, running them posteriorly to mimic the direction of gluteal fibers (figure 8.10a).

■ Tape the lateral side of the knee joint. This is a temporary measure usually used to address knee pain. It can be useful in providing sensory feedback to clients but will have little if any impact on anatomical (rather than postural) genu varum. One approach is to tape as if for a lateral collateral ligament sprain where your aim is to prevent further gapping of the lateral side of the knee. In this case you would attach a horizontal fixing strip above and below the knee and then make a cross shape between them, using two further tapes, aiming for the centre of the cross to fall over the lateral collateral ligament (figure 8.10b). Some therapists tape with the client standing, but it can be helpful to position the client in side lying with the affected knee uppermost. In this way gravity helps reduce the gapping on the lateral side of the knee before taping.

■ Consider the value of myofascial release using techniques such as the cross-hand over the medial aspect of the knee.

■ Passively stretch internal rotators of the hip, using the ideas put forward in chapter 7 for internal rotation of the hip.

■ Passively stretch additional muscles you identify as tight, using table 8.4 as a guide. This could include the quadriceps and the adductors (figure 8.10c).

■ Massage shortened muscles with the view to lengthening them. Note that when you massage the adductors, it can be uncomfortable to treat them with your client in the supine position, which sometimes tenses the lateral side of the knee, so a side-lying position can be preferable (figure 8.10d).

■ Consider referring your client to a physiotherapist or sport therapist for specialist balance training.

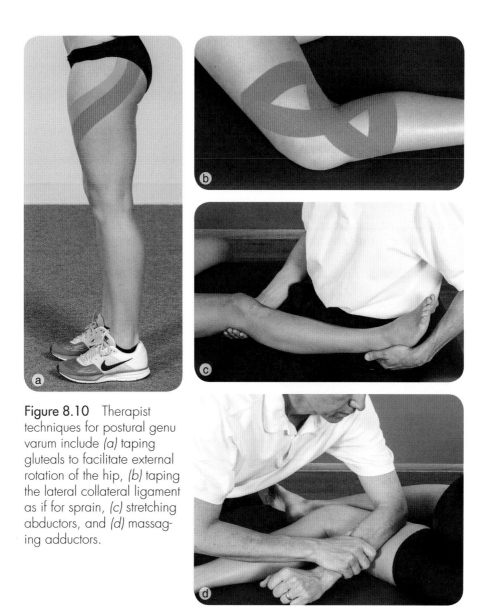

Figure 8.10 Therapist techniques for postural genu varum include *(a)* taping gluteals to facilitate external rotation of the hip, *(b)* taping the lateral collateral ligament as if for sprain, *(c)* stretching abductors, and *(d)* massaging adductors.

What Your Client Can Do

- Identify lazy standing postures that aggravate the genu varum stance. This sometimes occurs when tired and in the habit of shifting weight onto one leg.

- Actively stretch internal rotators of the hip. One of the challenges in doing this is that the kinds of stretches usually advocated for these muscles (e.g., figure 8.3b) promote gapping of the lateral side of the knee, so they need to be performed with care.

- Strengthen external hip rotators using exercises such as prone hip extension and bridging.

- Stretch hip adductors, taking care not to strain the outside of the knee.

- Consider wearing a knee brace when taking part in sporting activities. This may alleviate pain during weight bearing and may lessen the chances of injury.

- If possible, avoid sports that involve high-impact or excessive loading because this increases stress through the knee joint, further compressing and tensing structures

- Where these have been found to be lengthened, strengthen tibialis posterior and the long toe flexors. One method is to use a soft stretchy band, fairly wide, and use the toes (not the ankle) to stretch it (figure 8.11).

- Consider using orthotics to correct foot pronation as recommended by a podiatrist.

- To correct postural bowlegs, Kendall and colleagues (1993) advocate standing with the feet about 5 centimeters apart, knees comfortably relaxed, then tightening the buttock muscles to experience a lifting of the arches of the feet. Transfer a slight amount of weight onto the lateral sides of the feet, then tighten the buttocks further in an attempt to rotate the legs slightly outward and have the patellae facing forwards.

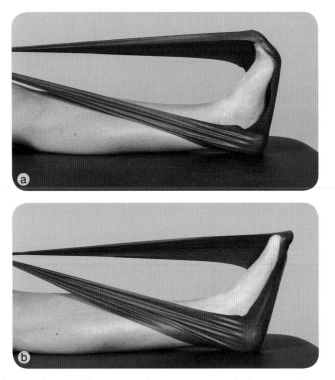

Figure 8.11 Client techniques for postural genu varum include strengthening of tibialis posterior and long toe flexors where these are found to be lengthened by placing a stretchy band along the underside of the foot and using the toes to stretch the band.

Genu Valgum

The normal angle formed between the anatomical axis of the femur and the anatomical axis of the tibia on the medial side of the knee is approximately 195 degrees (Levangie and Norkin 2001). Popularly termed *knock knees*, genu valgum is misalignment of the knee joint such that the medial tibiofemoral angle is *greater than* 195 degrees (figure 8.12a). The severity of the posture is revealed by observing the distance between the medial malleoli when a patient stands with the medial femoral condyles touching (figure 8.12b). Valgus deformity can occur unilaterally (figure 8.12c).

An increase in in the valgus angle of the knee often coincides with leg length discrepancy, occurring on the side where the leg is longer, and there is also posterior pelvic torsion of the ilium on that side (Cooperstein and Lew 2009).

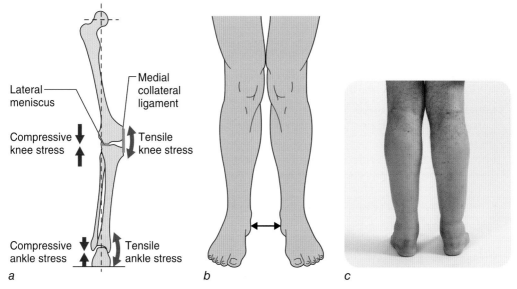

Lateral meniscus

Medial collateral ligament

Compressive knee stress

Tensile knee stress

Compressive ankle stress

Tensile ankle stress

a   b   c

Figure 8.12 *(a)* Genu valgum, showing tensile and compressive forces in the genu varum posture. Note the gapping of the knee joint in genu valgum posture, with increased tension on the medial collateral ligament and compression of the lateral meniscus. When a patient stands with medial femoral condyles touching, the degree of valgus deformity can be assessed by *(b)* observing the distance between the medial malleoli. *(c)* Unilateral genu valgum of the right knee.

TIP The iliotibial band may be shortened. In this posture the lateral side of the foot is elevated from the floor. Fibularis muscles are shortened where there is eversion of the foot, but sometimes the foot position changes to compensate for genu valgum, so you could find excessive subtalar supination. There may be discomfort in the tibiofibular joint as the result of compression of lateral knee structures in this posture.

Consequences of Genu Valgum

In the genu valgum posture there is increased tensile stress in the medial side of the knee and ankle and increased compressive forces on the lateral side of the knee and ankle (figure 8.12a).

In this posture, gapping occurs at the medial side of the joint, increasing tension on the medial collateral ligament (figure 8.12a), which could become weakened, providing less stability for the knee and increasing the likelihood of medial collateral ligament injury. The lateral meniscus is compressed, possibly causing damage here too.

During normal bilateral weight bearing, forces are transmitted via the mechanical axis of the knee, through the centre of the knee joint, and distributed equally through the medial and lateral compartments. In the genu valgum posture, force is shifted to the lateral aspect of the knee and could affect balance and gait. Altered joint mechanics may predispose a patient to knee pathology. Malalignment is associated with higher rates of knee osteoarthritis (McWilliams et al. 2010).

Gracilis, semitendinosus, and sartorius are all lengthened and tensioned. Tensor fasciae latae and the iliotibial band are compressed, as are tissues of the lateral leg compartment (see table 8.5).

The abnormal joint position is also likely to affect the normal glide and roll of the femur on the tibia that occur during flexion and extension movements of the knee. There may also be a tendency for the patella to be pulled laterally, which could disrupt this bone's normal gliding mechanism. Together these altered joint mechanics are likely to compromise knee function. In extreme cases the genu valgum posture could contribute to degenerative changes in the patellofemoral joint. Proprioception is likely to be altered, which could affect balance.

Genu valgum is associated with postural change in other joints. This includes lumbar spine rotation on the contralateral side and excessive adduction and medial rotation of the hip, lateral tibial torsion, inversion of the talus, supination of the subtalar or intertarsal joints and pes planus (Riegger-Krugh and Keysor 1996).

Table 8.5 Muscle Lengths Associated With Genu Valgum Knee Posture

Area	Shortened muscles	Lengthened muscles
Thigh	Biceps femoris relative to semi-membranosus and semitendinosus Tensor fasciae latae Hip adductors	Gracilis Semimembranosus and semi-tendinosus relative to biceps femoris Sartorius
Leg	Fibulari (peroneals)	

What You Can Do as a Therapist

- Consider referring your client to a podiatrist, who may be able to offer specialist advice. For example, angled insoles can be used to transfer the load from the lateral to the medial compartment of the knee and perhaps alter the tibiofemoral angle. Use of medial wedge insoles has been found to reduce pain and improve function in patients with valgus knee osteoarthritis (Rodrigues et al. 2008).

- Passively stretch the iliotibial band using techniques such as stretching (figure 8.13a) and massage.

- Use myofascial release to release the band, or use soft tissue release (figure 8.13b).

- Use static pressures to tensor fasciae latae to address any trigger points found in this muscle and to encourage relaxation and lengthening of the tissue (figure 8.2d).

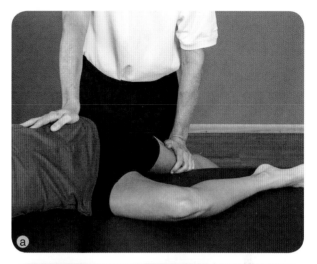

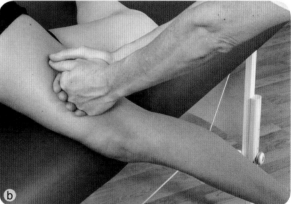

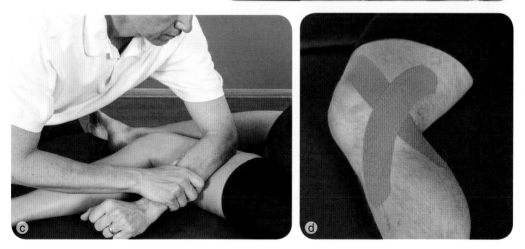

Figure 8.13 Therapist techniques for genu valgum include (a) stretching of the ITB, (b) soft tissue release to the ITB, (c) massage to the gracilis, and (d) taping the medial side of the knee.

- Massage gracilis where this is found to be shortened. If you choose to treat your client in the side-lying position with the client resting on the affected limb, the adductors will be accessible yet the knee is supported by the couch (figure 8.13c), and you can massage the gracilis without the risk of gapping the knee joint further.

- Tape the medial side of the knee joint, but note that this is a temporary measure usually used for overcoming pain and will not provide long-term correction of a genu valgum knee. One way to apply tape is as if you were taping a medial collateral sprain, attempting to orientate the centre of a cross over the medial collateral ligament (figure 8.13d). A tip here is to position your client in side lying, resting on the affected limb. In this way the medial collateral ligament will be uppermost but the knee will be supported by the couch, and you can apply gentle pressure as you apply the tape, taking the knee into a more neutral position, providing this is comfortable for the client.

- Use passive stretching and massage to help lengthen shortened tissues in the leg, such as the fibulari.

What Your Client Can Do

- Identify and avoid lazy standing postures that aggravate the genu valgum stance. This sometimes occurs when tired or in the habit of shifting weight onto one leg. Avoid resting the feet around chair legs when sitting (figure 8.3a) because this strains the medial side of the knee and ankle.

- Actively stretch the adductor and abductor muscles of the hip. Tensor fasciae latae and the iliotibial band may be shortened, but the hip falls into adduction in the genu valgum posture, so you will need to assess hip muscles and guide your client on which are shortened and may need stretching. Stretching the adductors with the knee flexed may be preferable to long-leg stretching, which could aggravate the valgus posture. Using a tennis ball to trigger and stretch tensor fasciae latae can be useful but in practice can be a difficult position for many clients to achieve without compromising the knee joint in the process (figure 7.15c). One solution is to tape the knee joint before the client attempts to use the ball or for the client to wear a knee brace whilst using the ball.

- Use a foam roller to address tension in the iliotibial band (figure 7.15d). Osteoporotic clients should not use this because it places considerable pressure on the lateral thigh. Although reported anecdotally to be useful by runners and those engaged in regular sports, it is difficult for many clients to use, so exercise extreme care so as not to use the roller on the knee joint itself.

- If possible, avoid sports that involve high impact because this increases stress through the knee joint, further compressing and tensing structures.

- A knee brace is an option. Note that this may alleviate pain during weight bearing but will not redress bony structures.

- Orthotics are an option for correcting foot pronation, if recommended by a podiatrist.

Tibial Torsion

True tibial torsion is twisting of the tibia within the bone itself, around its longitudinal axis. With respect to the proximal end, the distal end of the tibia is twisted laterally and contributes to the toe-out posture observed in normal standing. There is no agreed norm for the degree of twist because studies have used different proximal and distal end points on the tibia when making measurements. One method of measurement is to take either MRI or CT scans of the proximal (figure 8.14a) and distal (figure 8.14b) ends of the tibia, just below and above the articulating surfaces, respectively, then draw lines bisecting each scan. The tibial torsion angle is the angle formed by the bisecting lines (figure 8.14c).

In their review of nine studies carried out between 1909 and 1975, Turner and Smillie (1981) report tibial torsion measurements ranging from 14 to 23 degrees but note that different measuring devices were used, making comparison difficult. In a more recent study, Strecker and colleagues (1997) record torsion in 504 normal tibiae as 34.9 ± 15.9 degrees. Levangie and Norkin (2001) suggest using the figure of 20 to 30 degrees for tibial torsion in the normal population.

Assessing tibial torsion before treatment is a challenge. Not only are there differences in the degree of tibial torsion between different studies, but different degrees of torsion have been found between the left and right tibiae of the same patients (Strecker et al. 1997; Gandhi et al. 2014) and among ethnic groups. For example, Mullaji and

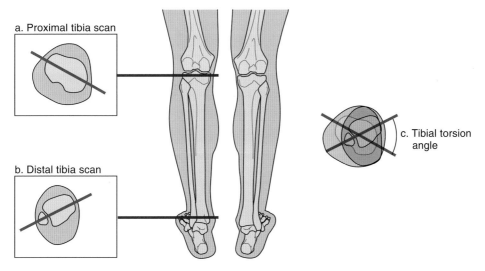

Figure 8.14 One method for calculating true tibial torsion, using the left leg as an example: (a) Scan of proximal tibia, just distal to the articulating surface. (Note the absence of the fibula at this point of cross-section.) (b) Distal tibia, just superior to the articulating surface. The fibula can be seen as the smaller bone because it is present at this level of cross-section. (c) Tibial torsion angle.

colleagues (2008) recorded tibial torsion in 100 limbs of only 21.6 ± 7.6 degrees in a study of non-arthritic Indian adults. Mullaji and colleagbues suggest that the variation between groups could be due to culture-specific sitting postures. For example, Japanese people traditionally sit on the floor in knee flexion, with the feet turned inwards and buttocks resting on the feet, exerting an *internal* force on the tibia, whereas sitting cross-legged, as is common in some Indian populations (the lotus position in yoga), increases *external* tibial rotation.

In a clinical setting tibial torsion tends to refer to torsion of the leg (i.e., rotation between the tibia and femur at the knee joint and movement between the tibia and talus at the ankle joint). Whether torsion is pure (within the bone itself irrespective of joints) or clinical (longitudinal rotation about the leg due to lower-limb joint positions or true torsion), it is difficult to identify purely from postural assessment. A good starting point is to observe your client from the front and to note where the tibial tuberosities lie. Are they facing forwards and symmetrical, or does one face inwards (internal tibial torsion) or outwards (external tibial torsion)? Observe the position of the feet. Internal tibial torsion is associated with a toe-in posture and external torsion with a toe-out posture.

However, a patient can appear to have normal tibiae when in fact these are torsioned. An example is in figure 8.15. At first glance the patient's legs appear normal because her left and right tibial tuberosities are facing forwards. But observe her right knee, which does not face forwards. This indicates internal rotation of the femur. With an internal rotation of the femur you would expect to also have in-toeing, yet the client's feet are facing forwards. In order for the feet to face forwards, the tibia would have had to torsion *externally*. A way of testing whether there is external rotation is to ask your client to stand so that the

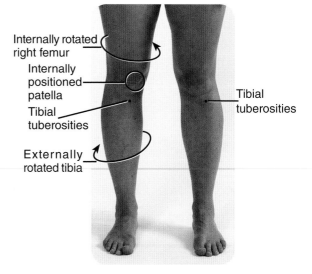

Figure 8.15 Patient with external tibial torsion of the right leg, which at first glance appears normal.

knees are facing forwards, if able. When a patient with external tibial torsion stands with the knees facing forwards, the external tibial torsion will be much more marked because the feet will have been placed in a marked toe-out position.

Although not all studies agree, some have found that torsion varies between the left and right legs within the same individual, with greater outward rotation of the right leg compared to the left (Clementz 1988; Mullaji et al. 2008). It is not clear why this is.

Consequences of Internal Tibial Torsion

During walking, the pelvis rotates about the weight-bearing hip joint, with the pelvis on the side of the swinging leg moving forward. Various segments of the leg rotate in the same direction as the pelvis and in phase with pelvic rotation. The amplitude of rotation increases proximally to distally, with the tibia rotating about its long axis three times as much as the pelvis rotates (Inman 1966). Rotation of this kind is therefore a normal part of gait, so excessive internal or external rotation will adversely affect these biomechanics and is likely to increase the energy expenditure of walking.

Some muscles have the ability to affect joints they do not cross. Although the mechanisms for this are unclear, it could be due to the interconnectedness of muscles synched via the fascial system. Gluteals and soleus can each affect both the hip and the knee joints. Excessive tibial torsion has been found to reduce the capacity of these muscles and, as a result, diminish hip and knee extension during gait (Hicks et. al 2007).

Certain sports might aggravate this posture. For example, golfers develop postures throughout their bodies that are associated with rotation, including in the joints of the lower limbs and in the soft tissues associated with these. The pivoting movement inherent to golf increases the likelihood of tibial torsion on the leg that remains static. For example, taking the club to the right at the start of a swing and rotating the upper body clockwise to the right produce internal rotation of the left hip and internal torsion on the right leg, which is fixed to the ground.

Torsion of the tibia alters the position of the menisci with respect to the femur and the direction of pull of the patella. Ultimately it affects how forces are transmitted through the knee joint. These could be reasons why tibial torsion is associated with early-onset arthritis, patellofemoral arthritis, genu valgum and genu varum. Malalignment of the knee joint could increase the risk of knee injury.

Clinical tibial torsion also affects the feet and ankles (see table 8.6). Lateral tibial torsion is associated with a toe-out foot position and increased supination, heel inversion and accentuation of the medial longitudinal arch. Medial tibial torsion is associated with a toe-in foot position, which can lead to feelings of clumsiness when walking or actual tripping. There is increased subtalar pronation, the heel is everted and the medial longitudinal arch is decreased. These changes may cause pain, reduce balance and affect gait. Abnormal joint positions in the foot and ankle are likely to impair sporting performance and in some cases could contribute to early joint degeneration, especially in in sports or occupations involving repeated high impact. In a study of 836 patients, Turner and Smillie (1981) found that external torsion of the tibia was correlated with those patients who had lesions of the extensor apparatus, notably unstable patellofemoral joints and Osgood-Schlatter disease. It is not known whether these conditions lead to the development of increased external tibial torsion or whether pre-existing increased tibial torsion predisposed the patients to subsequent development of patellofemoral instability and Osgood-Schlatter. By contrast, patients with everted feet (associated with internal tibial torsion) have an advantage when running distances of 15 to 20 meters because this posture promotes

(continued)

Consequences of Internal Tibial Torsion *(continued)*

short, rapid steps, theoretically because tibial torsion shortens the hamstrings, limiting a wider step. There is greater ground contact whilst moving, and this may improve dynamic balance (Bloomfield et al. 1994).

Because tibial torsion can affect and be affected by movements in the pelvis, hip, foot and ankle, there may be imbalance in muscles throughout the entire lower limb, and these will be highly individualized. Muscles shown in table 8.6 provide a guide only. Because of the small degree of rotational movement involved in tibial torsion, there are few significant changes to the length of muscles in this posture. Joint position and the effect on ligaments and articular structures may be of greater significance than muscle lengths. It is likely that many structures contribute to the checking of knee rotation, including the cruciates, collateral ligaments, posteromedial capsule, posterolateral capsule and popliteus tendon, and menisci distorted in the direction of the corresponding femoral condyle (Levangie and Norkin 2001). These structures will be affected when there is an increase in torsion involving joints (rather than pure torsion within the tibia). The degree of change in the muscles listed in table 8.7 may be minor and are included only to show that some change is likely to occur, as, for example, the distal attachments of the hamstrings are re-orientated as the tibia rotates either internally or externally.

Table 8.6 Tibial Torsion and Corresponding Changes in Foot

	Lateral tibial torsion	Medial tibial torsion
Foot position	Toe-out	Toe-in
Foot changes	Increased subtalar supination	Increased subtalar pronation
	Inversion of heel	Eversion of heel
	Accentuation of medial longitudinal arch	Decrease in medial longitudinal arch

Table 8.7 Muscle Lengths Associated With Increased Tibial Torsion

Direction of torsion	Shortened muscles	Lengthened muscles
External tibial torsion	Biceps femoris relative to semitendinosus and semimembranosus Iliotibial band Sartorius Muscles and ligaments associated with pronation of the foot	Semitendinosus and semimembranosus relative to biceps femoris Popliteus Muscles and ligaments associated with pronation of the foot
Internal tibial torsion	Semitendinosus and semimembranosus relative to biceps femoris Popliteus Muscles and ligaments associated with supination of the foot	Biceps femoris relative to semitendinosus and semimembranosus Sartorius Iliotibial band Muscles and ligaments associated with supination of the foot

What You Can Do as a Therapist

Hands-on therapies could be useful in addressing clinical tibial torsion—by promoting correct joint alignment at the hip, knee, ankle and foot—whereas they cannot be used to correct true tibial torsion. This section focuses on the correction of clinical tibial torsion.

- Acknowledge that where the postural asymmetries you observe are the result of true tibial torsion, non-surgical intervention is ineffective.

- Help your client to identify and avoid occasions when posture may aggravate tibial torsion.

- Refer to a podiatrist who may be able to advise on whether orthotics would be beneficial for your client.

- Tape the tibia into a more neutral position but recognize that this is a temporary measure only. Spiral your tape across the front of the knee as shown in figure 8.16, taking it diagonally behind the knee and onto and across the thigh.

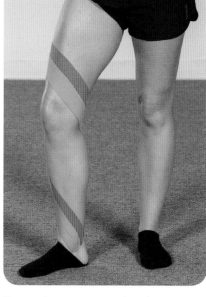

Figure 8.16 Taping the tibia is a temporary technique to alleviate symptoms associated with internal tibial torsion.

- Address any muscle imbalance you find at the hip, ankle and foot and provide your client with any necessary stretches or exercises they can use to help correct these imbalances. The sections on feet may be of particular interest.

What Your Client Can Do

- Avoid postures that contribute to tibial torsion. For example, sleeping in the prone position encourages internal tibial torsion, as does sitting on the feet Japanese style, so clients with internal tibial torsion should avoid these. However, could these positions be used to promote internal torsion for clients with *external* tibial torsion? Conversely, sitting in a W position encourages external tibial torsion. Could it be used to encourage external torsion in clients with *internal* tibial torsion?

- Theoretically, clients engaged in sports with a high rotatory component (e.g., golf, shot put, javelin) would benefit from trying to work both sides of the body equally. This is unlikely to be practical because people have a tendency to favor one side of the body and display side-specific skills often developed over many years of practice. So trying to replicate the movement on the non-dominant side of the body in order to achieve the same results is unrealistic.

- Consider wearing a brace or orthotics where these have been recommended by a specialist.

- Address any muscle imbalance you find at the hip, ankle and foot. The section on feet may be of particular interest.

Pes Planus

Commonly termed *flatfoot*, pes planus is loss of the normal longitudinal plantar arch, giving the foot a flattened appearance (figure 8.17c). When present in both weight-bearing and non-weight-bearing positions it is known as *rigid flatfoot*. When the arch is absent in standing but present in non-weight-bearing positions, it is termed *flexible flatfoot*. In this posture there is excessive pronation as the talus glides medially over the calcaneus and comes into contact with the ground. This is reflected by the shape of the footprint (figure 8.17d), which shows greater surface area than normal because a greater portion of the sole is in contact with the ground. The flattened appearance of the foot makes this an easy posture to identify in a patient (figure 8.17e).

Pes planus is when the navicular bone (figure 8.17c) lies beneath the Feiss line, a line running from the top of the medial malleolus to the base of the first metatarsal (in the normal foot, figure 8.17a).

In addition to flattening of the foot, when you observe your client from behind you may notice that the toes drift outward and the ankle appears to fall inwards as the calcaneus pronates (the pes valgus ankle posture). Pes planus is considered mild where hindfoot valgus is 4 to 6 degrees, moderate where it is 6 to 10 degrees, and severe where it is 10 to 15 degrees (Magee 2002). For more information on calcaneal pronation, see the section on the pes valgus posture.

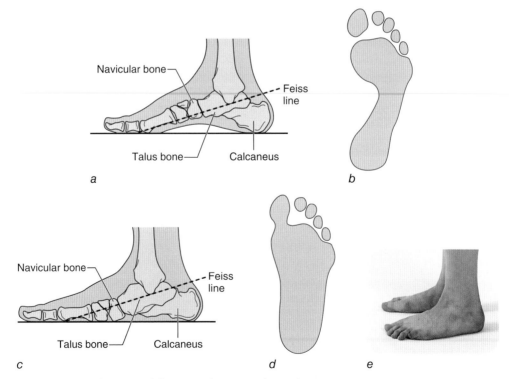

Figure 8.17 (a, b) Normal foot; (c, d, e) pes planus foot.

TIP In addition to lengthening of muscles, there is overstretching of ligaments and of the plantar fascia.

Consequences of Pes Planus

The arch of the foot provides a spring mechanism essential for helping to absorb and dissipate forces during gait. Loss of the arch means reduced shock absorption, which could contribute to the development of stress injuries to the feet, ankles and bones of the leg. In some cases this posture could impair balance and stability. However, studies carried out using military personnel do not support the notion of increased incidence of injury in patients with flat feet.

During the mid-stance of gait the foot pronates slightly via the talus and goes into slight supination during push-off. The tibia responds to these movements by rotating internally and then externally. A talus that is incorrectly placed or does not function optimally therefore hinders tibial function and affects the entire kinetic chain of the lower limb. The gait of a patient with pes planus has been described as slouchy and jarring, with exaggerated flexion of the knee and weight bearing on the heel such that the demands of muscular activity are increased (Whitman 2010). An increase in tension in the muscles of the feet whilst walking has been found in patients with pes planus, which could explain why people with flat feet have more pain when they walk for long periods (Fan et al. 2011).

People with flexible flatfoot are more likely to have hammertoes and overlapping toes (Hagedorn et al. 2013). These can cause discomfort and difficulty wearing certain types of footwear.

Individuals with severe pes planus have pain. In addition to pain in the heel, arch and ankle and along the outside of the foot there may be pain in the shinbone and even low back, hip or knee (American College of Foot and Ankle Surgeons 2014a). There may be pain and swelling of the tibialis posterior tendon and pain not only in activities such as running but also in walking or standing (American Academy of Orthopedic Surgeons 2014).

The pes planus foot posture stretches and weakens the plantar aponeurosis and the intrinsic muscles of the foot and ligaments. Patients with hypermobility syndromes who already have increased laxity in the ligaments of the foot may have pain in the foot, ankle and leg as well as weakness (Tinkle 2008).

Specimens of tibialis posterior tendon taken from patients with adult-acquired flatfoot reveal the presence of enzymes that break down and weaken the tendon (Corps et al. 2012). Dysfunction of the posterior tibial tendon results in relative internal rotation of the tibia and talus and a flattening of the medial arch. Over time this contributes to deformity of the ankle, eventually leading the calcaneus to impinge against the fibula, causing pain (Myerson 1996).

Table 8.8 Muscle Lengths Associated With Pes Planus

	Shortened muscles	Lengthened muscles
Deep	n/a	Intrinsic plantar muscles Tendon of tibialis posterior Long muscles of sole of foot
Superficial	Fibulari due to excessive pronation	n/a

What You Can Do as a Therapist

- Recognize that where flatfoot is due to structural abnormality and is rigid, hands-on therapy is ineffective. The main focus of your treatment for flexible flatfoot is on the prevention of excessive pronation when the foot is loaded and this is achieved by controlling valgus (eversion) of the calcaneus (Levangie and Norkin 2001). Refer to the pes valgus section of this book.

- Refer your client to a podiatrist who may be able to offer advice on the use of orthotics. There is moderate evidence that they may improve function and the energy cost of walking but only low level evidence that they improve pain, reduce rearfoot eversion, alter loading and impact forces and reduce rearfoot eversion and inversion movements (Banwell et al. 2014).

- Be aware that changes made to the position of bones of the foot affect not only the lower limb but the entire kinetic chain throughout the body. Your client may experience either a relief or an exacerbation of symptoms elsewhere as a result of treatments to the foot.

- Popularly known as foot gymnastics, foot dexterity exercises are sometimes advocated to help strengthen the intrinsic muscles of the foot. However, these have not been shown to be effective over and above general exercise (Hartman et al. 2009).

- Teach your client exercises to strengthen plantar flexors of the foot such as rising onto the toes.

- Address altered postures throughout the lower limb referring to the relevant sections in this book.

What Your Client Can Do

- One way to treat pes planus due to faulty postural activity of foot muscles is to rotate the legs outwards whilst keeping the feet on the floor (Perkins 1947). To better explain this to your client, you may wish to practice this yourself to see if you can feel your arch rising. Standing barefoot, consciously lift the medial arches by contracting your buttock muscles.

- Strengthen the intrinsic muscles of the foot with exercises such as using the toes to pick up a pencil or scrunch up a towel.

- Some clients find it fun to try foot gymnastics, which are commonly prescribed for flexible pes planus despite the evidence for their effectiveness being poor. Examples of the kinds of exercises used in foot gymnastics are using the feet and toes to tie a knot in a rope, using the toes to pick up and fasten a clothes peg to a line or to the edge of a cup, passing a stick or pencil back and forth with a partner, holding a paper cup between the toes of one foot and using the toes of the other foot to pick up small objects and deposit these in the cup, and using the toes to pick up small hoops and place them over a pole.

- Practice balancing as normal and on tiptoe.

- Walk barefoot (where this is safe) on various surfaces such as soil, sand or grass.

- The American College of Foot an Ankle Surgeons (2014b) recommend a reduction in prolonged walking and standing as well as a reduction in body weight in patients who are overweight, although this advice may be aimed more at helping to reduce the pain associated with this posture rather than postural correction.

- Where the flatfoot is the result of tibialis posterior dysfunction, wear flat, lace-up footwear that can accommodate orthosis where these have been recommended by a podiatrist (Kohls-Gatzoulis et al. 2004).

Pes Caves

In the pes caves posture (high arches), the calcaneus is supinated and the plantar arch is higher than normal (figure 8.18c) compared to the normal foot (figure 8.18a). Usually there is a varus (inverted) hindfoot, plantarflexed first metatarsal, adducted forefoot and claw toes (Burns et al. 2007). Footprints of a patient with pes cavus reveal reduced contact points with the ground (figure 8.18d) compared to footprints of a patient with normal feet (figure 8.18b). In observing this posture, look for claw toes, splaying of the forefoot and raised arch. Posteriorly you may observe that the calcaneus is supinated (pes varus).

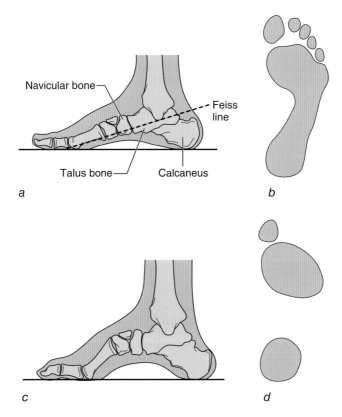

Figure 8.18 *(a, b)* Normal foot and *(c, d)* pes cavus foot with their associated footprints.

TIP With the longitudinal arch raised, each end of the arch is brought closer together and there is shortening of the plantar fascia.

Consequences of Pes Cavus Posture

There is increased pressure on the ball of the foot. It is suggested that patients with pes cavus foot posture may have hammertoes or claw toes; calluses on the ball, side or heel of the foot; pain when standing or walking; and an increased likelihood of ankle sprains due to the heel tilting inward (supinating) (American College of Foot and Ankle Surgeons 2014a).

Individuals with pes cavus sometimes have difficulty getting footwear to fit and have reduced tolerance for walking (Burns et al. 2007). Runners with high arches report a greater incidence of ankle injuries, bony injuries and lateral injuries (Williams et al. 2001).

There may be painful calluses beneath the metatarsal heads caused by loss of the metatarsal arch and maybe osteoarthritic changes in the tarsal region (Magee 2002).

Where the subtalar and transverse tarsal joints are locked into supination, this will prevent shock absorption, and the hindfoot supination may cause rotational stress on the leg (Levangie and Norkin 2001). As with pes planus, an alteration in foot function has an effect on the entire kinetic chain of the lower limb.

Table 8.9   Muscle Lengths Associated With Pes Caves

	Shortened muscles	Lengthened muscles
Superficial	Where there are claw toes, associated toe extensor tendons are short	n/a
Deep	Shortening of intrinsic foot muscles	n/a

What You Can Do as a Therapist

- Recognize that where pes cavus is the result of a neurological condition, hands-on therapy will be ineffective. Some studies have shown that there is no evidence for the effectiveness of any treatments for the pes cavus posture other than orthotics (Burns et al. 2007).

- Consider referring your client to a podiatrist. Orthotics, shoe modifications and bracing may be helpful (American College of Foot and Ankle Surgeons 2014a). Custom-made orthotics have been shown to provide significant benefit (Burns et al. 2007).

- Be aware that changes made to the position of bones of the foot affect not only the lower limb but the entire kinetic chain throughout the body. Your client may have either a relief or an exacerbation of symptoms elsewhere as a result of treatments to the foot.

- Stretching of gastrocnemius has been advocated as a useful non-surgical intervention for pes cavus (Manoli et al. 2005).

- Address altered postures throughout the lower limb, referring to the relevant sections in this book.

- Although stretching of the plantar fascia with massage (figure 8.19a) and passive dorsiflexion of the toes (figure 8.19b) may provide some pain relief, there is little evidence to show that it affects pes cavus foot posture.

- Refer to the section on pes varus for the correction of calcaneal supination.

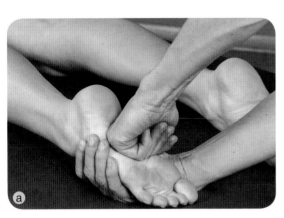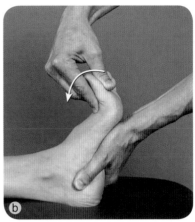

Figure 8.19 Therapist techniques for pes cavus such as *(a)* stretching of the soft tissues of the plantar surface of the foot with massage and *(b)* passive dorsiflexion of the toes will theoretically help lengthen these tissues, but their effectiveness is unsubstantiated.

What Your Client Can Do

- Consider wearing orthotics or a brace and having alterations made to the shoes if this has been recommended by a podiatrist (American College of Foot and Ankle Surgeons 2014a).

- Theoretically, active toe extension stretches (figure 8.20*a* and *b*) and use of a ball (figure 8.20*c*) to stretch the plantar fascia will help lengthen soft tissues, but the effectiveness of such exercises is unsubstantiated.

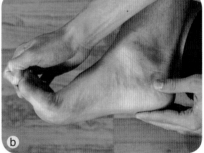

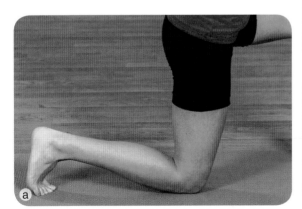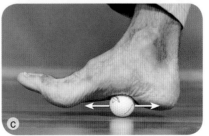

Figure 8.20 Client techniques for pes cavus such as *(a)* stretching of the soft tissues of the plantar surface of the foot with active toe extension and *(b)* stretches and *(c)* use of a ball rolled over the sole theoretically help lengthen these tissues, but the effectiveness of such exercises is unsubstantiated.

Pes Valgus

Pes is a term restricted to any deformity of the foot of acquired origin, and *valgus* refers to bones distal to the joint moving in a single plane away from the midline (Ritchie and Keim 1964). In the pes valgus foot posture (pronated foot), the calcaneus is the bone that moves away from the midline and is often described as being *abducted* (figure 8.21*b*). Another way to describe the pes valgus posture is that there is eversion (or valgus) of the heel. There is pronation of the foot and the medial longitudinal arch is reduced in height.

The posture is easy to identify because in normal foot posture, the lateral malleolus is positioned slightly inferior to the medial malleolus, whereas in the pes valgus posture the lateral malleolus lies even lower. Your client may appear to be bearing weight more on the medial side of the heel (often evidenced by increased wear on the sole of the shoe) with less pressure on the lateral side of the heel. When assessing a client, it can sometimes be helpful to imagine a line through the tibia, talus and calcaneus, which in the normal foot posture is vertical but deviates in the pes valgus posture, forming an obtuse angle on the lateral side of the ankle.

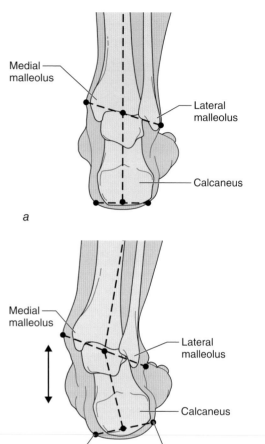

Figure 8.21 *(a)* Normal foot posture and *(b)* pes valgus foot posture noting tensile and compressive stresses.

Consequences of Pes Valgus

In the pes valgus posture there are increased tensile stresses on the medial side of the ankle and increased compressive stresses on the lateral side of the ankle (figure 8.21*b*). Anatomic foot type does not appear to be a risk factor for ankle sprains (Beynnon et al. 2002) (although many studies tested participants standing barefoot and not dynamically). Nevertheless, theoretically, increased tensile stress on the medial side of the ankle could lengthen and weaken the medial collateral (deltoid) ligament, predisposing a patient to medial collateral ankle sprain.

Ligaments between the tibia and fibula contribute to the function of both superior and inferior tibiofibular joints (Levangie and Norkin 2001). Compressive stress on the lateral side of the ankle could therefore affect the proper functioning not only of the distal tibiofibular joint but of the proximal tibiofibular joint too.

A pronated foot increases the likelihood of having hallux valgus and overlapping toes (Hagedorn et al. 2013) as well as metatarsalgia, interdigital neuritis, and plantar fasciitis (Fowler 2004).

Table 8.10 illustrates muscle length changes associated with this posture. Such changes may explain why the pronated foot requires more muscle work for maintaining stance stability than the supinated foot (Magee 2002) and why there may be myositis or tendinitis of tibialis anterior and tibialis posterior (Fowler 2004). People with pronated feet are more likely to have Achilles tendinitis or tendinosis due to greater demands placed on the tendon when walking (American College of Foot and Ankle Surgeons 2014b). Spindles in ankle muscles are significant for the control of posture and balance whilst walking (Sorensen et al. 2002). Muscles listed in table 8.10 all cross the ankle joint, and changes to their length or health are therefore likely to affect balance too. This could be particularly significant for older adults.

Fowler (2004) suggests that excessive foot pronation is associated with calcaneal bursitis and may contribute to medial knee injury, patellofemoral syndrome, iliotibial band syndrome, shin splints, trochanteric bursitis, anterior shift of the pelvis, and lumbar facet syndrome and sacrococcygeal dysfunction in the spine.

Patients with medial compartment knee osteoarthritis have been found to have a more pronated foot compared to controls (Levinger et al. 2010) and to walk with greater rearfoot eversion (Levinger et al. 2012) as in the pes valgus posture. It is not clear whether pes valgus develops in response to medial compartment knee osteoarthritis or whether the foot posture itself contributes to the development of this knee pathology. There may be pain in both the medial and lateral side of the talocrural joint (Gross 1995).

Proper arthrokinematic movement in the foot and ankle is essential for normal gait, and abnormal pronation results in the inability of the foot to absorb the forces of weight bearing effectively (Donatelli 1987). In this posture the heel abducts (everts). In the closed chain (weight bearing), this forces the talus to adduct and plantar flex. The tibia follows the motion of the talus and so is forced into slight internal rotation. Additionally there may be internal rotation of the femur and rotation of the pelvis (Riegger-Krugh and Keysor 1996). Pes valgus may be associated with the genu valgum (knock-knee) posture. Raising the lateral side of the foot (as in the pes valgus foot posture) results in significant changes in pelvic tilt and torsion (Betsch et al. 2011).

Given the changes in other joints of the lower limb associated with this posture, it is easy to see why it is popularly believed that pes valgus posture may be associated with an increased risk of injury. However, measurements of static lower-limb biomechanical alignment have not been found to be related to injury in recreational athletes (Lun et al. 2004).

Table 8.10   Muscle Lengths Associated With Pes Valgus

Area	Shortened muscles	Lengthened muscles
Ankle and leg	Fibulari (peroneals) Gastrocnemius Soleus	Tibialis posterior Adductor hallucis Flexor hallucis longus Flexor digitorum longus
Thigh	Where there are associated changes at the hip and knee: biceps femoris, hip adductors, tensor fasciae latae	Where there are associated changes at the hip and knee: gluteus maximus, gluteus medius

TIP In addition to shortening of muscles on the lateral side of the leg, there may be tightness in the iliotibial band.

What You Can Do as a Therapist

- Refer your client to a podiatrist. The use of orthotics to control the amount of pronation during the stance phase of gait, for example, has profound effects on pain and dysfunction in the lower extremity (Donatelli 1987).

- Taping is a popular intervention for the treatment of pes valgus. However, an experiment by Luque-Suarez and colleagues (2014) to see whether the application of kinesiotape helped correct excessive foot pronation found that it did not. Another study found that taping to correct pronation during walking and jogging was effective (Vicenzino et al. 2005).

- Apply passive stretches and massage to shortened muscles. For example, use soft tissue release on the evertor muscles with your client in a side-lying position (figures 8.22a) and stretch the calf with your client in the prone position (figure 8.22b), but take care to keep the ankle in a neutral position. This can be difficult, so lengthening of the tissues could be attempted through the application of deep tissue massage (figure 8.22c).

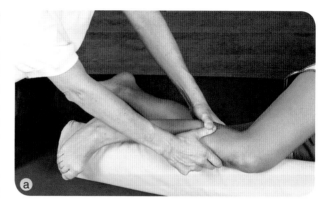

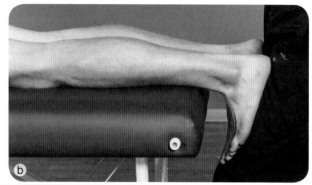

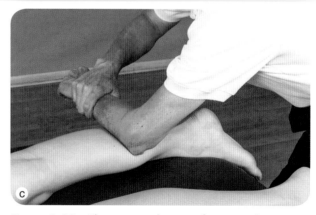

Figure 8.22 Therapist techniques for pes valgus include (a) soft tissue release to the fibulari muscles, (b) stretching and (c) massage of the calf.

- Address shortened muscles in the thigh where you find these.

- Use myofascial release to help release the whole of the lateral side of the lower limb.

- Help your client to strengthen ankle invertors.

- Identify whether gluteals are weakened muscles and help your client to strengthen these, perhaps via referral to an exercise professional.

What Your Client Can Do

- Recognize that self-treatment of pes valgus is limited.

- Consider wearing orthotics where these have been recommended by a podiatrist.

- Avoid resting the feet around chair legs when sitting because this pushes the feet into eversion. (figure 8.3a).

- Stretch shortened muscles such as the fibulari (figure 8.23a), gastrocnemius (figure 8.23b) and soleus (figure 8.23c). It is tempting to use a foam roller on fibulari, but this is not advised because it could damage the peroneal nerve as it passes around the head of the fibula where it is easily compressed.

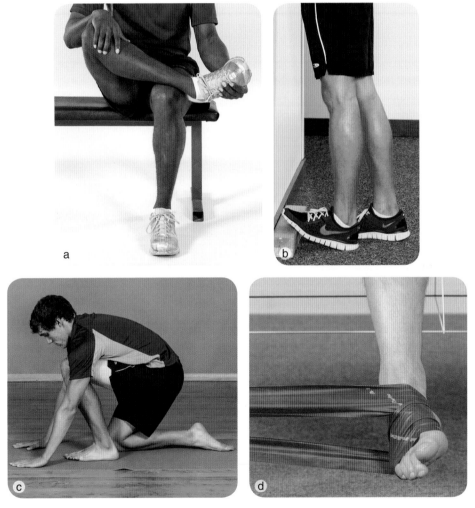

Figure 8.23 Client techniques for pes valgus include stretches to muscles that are shortened such as (a) fibulari, (b) gastrocnemius and (c) soleus and (d) strengthening exercise for ankle invertors.

- Stretch muscles of the hip and thigh, such as the hamstrings and adductors where these are found to be tight.
- Stretch the iliotibial band where this is found to be tight. One method is to use a foam roller, but take great care not to use the roller over the knee joint, and it is contraindicated for anyone with osteoporosis. Self-treat any trigger spots found here.
- Carry out exercises to strengthen ankle invertor muscles (figure 8.23d).
- Carry out exercises to strengthen weakened muscles of the hip, such as gluteals.

Pes Varus

Pes is a term restricted to any deformity of the foot of acquired origin, and the term *varus* means that bones distal to the joint move in a single plane towards the midline (Ritchie and Keim 1964). In the pes varus foot posture (supinated foot) the calcaneus is the bone that moves towards the midline and is often described as being adducted (figure 8.24b). Another way to describe the pes varus posture is to say that there is inversion (or varus) of the heel. There is supination of the foot, and the medial longitudinal arch may be accentuated.

In normal foot posture, the lateral malleolus is positioned slightly inferior to the medial malleolus (figure 8.24a), whereas in the pes varus posture the lateral malleolus lies higher, more parallel with the medial malleolus (figure 8.24b). Your client may appear to be bearing weight more on the lateral side of the heel, often evidenced by increased wear on the sole of the shoe, with less pressure on the medial side of the heel (figure 8.24b). When assessing a client, it can sometimes be helpful to imagine a line through the tibia, talus and calcaneus, which in the normal foot posture is vertical but deviates in the pes varus posture, forming an obtuse angle on the medial side of the ankle.

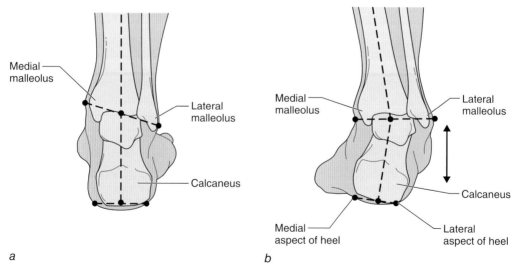

a *b*

Figure 8.24 (a) Normal foot posture and (b) pes varus foot posture noting compressive and tensile stresses.

TIP Plantar fascia on the sole of the foot is shortened.

Consequences of Pes Varus

There are increased compressive stress on the medial side of the ankle and increased tensile stresses on the lateral side of the ankle (figure 8.24). It is commonly believed that the pes varus posture predisposes a patient to ankle sprains, and this could be due to weakening of the lateral collateral ankle ligaments as a result of increased tensile stress. Review of the research into the relationship between foot type and lower-limb injury revels that anatomic foot type does not appear to be a risk factor for ankle sprains (Beynnon et al. 2002). However, many studies tested participants standing barefoot and not dynamically.

Increased tensile stress on the lateral side of the ankle could affect the proper functioning of the distal tibiofibular joint. Because both the distal and superior tibiofibular joints are linked, ligaments between the tibia and fibula contribute to the function of both joints (Levangie and Norkin 2001).

Table 8.11 illustrates muscle length changes associated with this posture. Spindles in ankle muscles are significant for the control of posture and balance whilst walking (Sorensen et al. 2002). Muscles listed in table 8.11 all cross the ankle joint; changes to their length or health are therefore likely to affect balance. This could be particularly significant for older adults. Further, in this posture the toes are lifted from the ground and often there is flexion of the big toe in an attempt to regain contact with the ground. It is essential that the toes function properly not just for balance but so that body weight can be distributed more evenly both in standing and whilst walking (Hughes et al. 1990).

You read in chapter 1 that in this posture the heel adducts (inverts). In the closed chain (weight bearing), this forces the talus to abduct and dorsiflex. As the tibia follows the motion of the talus, the tibia is then forced to externally rotate. This posture is also associated with external rotation of the femur and rotation of the pelvis (Riegger-Krugh and Keysor 1996). The consequences of this can be found in the section on tibial torsion.

Plantar fasciitis, heel spurs, Achilles tendinitis, metatarsalgia and calcaneal bursitis are developed in patients with excessive supination (Donatelli 1987).

As with pes valgus, changes in joints of the lower limb associated with this posture contribute to the popular belief that the pes varus posture may be associated with an increased risk of injury. Measurements of static lower-limb biomechanical alignment have not been found to be related to injury in recreational athletes (Lun et al. 2004). However, reviewing the research into predictive factors for lateral ankle sprains, Beynnon and colleagues (2002) report that increased hindfoot inversion (as is the case with an inverted heel) is a risk factor predisposing military trainees to lower-extremity overuse injury.

Table 8.11   Muscle Lengths Associated With Pes Varus

Area	Shortened muscles	Lengthened muscles
Foot	Flexor hallucis longus	Fibulari (peroneals)
	Flexor digitorum longus	Extensor digitorum longus
	Tibialis anterior	Extensor hallucis longus

What You Can Do as a Therapist

- Refer your client to a podiatrist. The use of orthotics to control the amount of supination during the stance phase of gait, for example, has profound effects on pain and dysfunction in the lower extremity (Donatelli 1987). The lateral side of the foot can be elevated with orthotics, but it is not clear whether this has a function in altering foot and ankle posture. Use of lateral wedge orthotics has been found to reduce symptoms in patients with medial compartment osteoarthritis at the knee (Malvankar et al. 2012) so may alter lower-limb posture. One of the challenges with this posture is that orthotics designed to correct foot supination can aggravate genu valgum where this is a corresponding posture.

- Massage and stretch shortened tissues, in this case on the plantar surface of the foot (8.19a), focusing on the medial side and the medial aspect of the ankle, taking care not to apply too much pressure. Positioning your client in side lying can be a useful treatment position for applying massage to the medial side of the leg (8.25a), and using a towel (figure 8.25b) or your thigh (figure 8.25c) can help you access and stretch tissues on the medial side of the ankle.

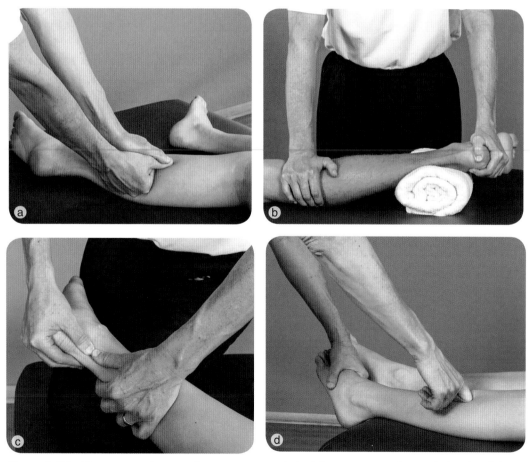

Figure 8.25 Therapist techniques for pes varus include (a) massage to the medial side of the leg, perhaps positioning the client with the medial side of the ankle uppermost using a (b) towel or (c) your thigh. (d) Massage to tibialis anterior.

- Tibialis anterior can be massaged (figure 8.25*d*).
- Use myofascial release to help release the whole of the medial side of the lower limb.
- Help your client to strengthen ankle evertors.

What Your Client Can Do

- Stretch the medial side of the foot and foot invertors by placing a small folded towel beneath the lateral side of the foot (figure 8.26*a*).
- Actively stretch flexor hallucis longus (figure 8.20*b*).
- Strengthen ankle evertors. One way to do this is by using a stretchy band placed around the foot and using the ankle evertors to stretch it (figure 8.26*b*).

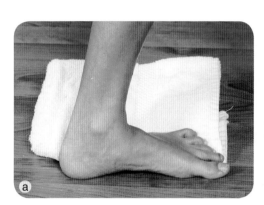 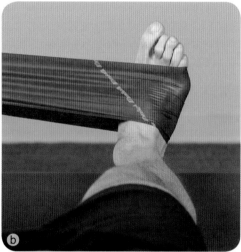

Figure 8.26 Client techniques for pes varus include *(a)* stretching the ankle invertor muscles by standing on a towel and *(b)* strengthening ankle evertors by placing a Theraband around the ankle and everting the foot.

Closing Remarks

In this chapter you learnt about 10 postures of the lower limb: internal rotation of the hip, genu recurvatum (knee hyperextension), genu flexum (knee flexion), genu varum (bow legs), genu valgum (knock knees), tibial torsion, flatfoot (pes planus), high arches in feet (pes caves), pronation in the foot (pes valgus) and supination in feet (pes varus). The anatomical features of each are stated along with photographic examples and illustrations. The consequences of each posture are described, and for each pathology a table contains lists of shortened and lengthened muscles that will help you plan your treatments. You learnt that changes in one part of the lower limb can affect parts both above and below it; therefore it is important to address the posture in those parts by referring to other sections of this book for ideas.

Correcting the Shoulder and Upper Limb

The six postures covered in part IV affect the shoulder and upper limb. Protracted scapula, internal rotation of the humerus, winged scapula and elevated shoulder are covered in chapter 9, Shoulder. Chapter 10, Elbow, describes how to treat flexed elbow and hyperextended elbow.

Shoulder

Learning outcomes

After reading this chapter, you should be able to do the following:

- List four postures common to the shoulder.
- Describe the anatomical features of each of these postures.
- Recognize these postures on a client.
- Give examples of the anatomical consequences of each posture.
- Name the muscles that are shortened and those that are lengthened in each posture.
- Give examples of appropriate treatments for the correction of each posture.
- Give the rationale for such treatments and state for which clients a particular treatment is contraindicated and why.
- Give examples of the kinds of stretches, exercises and activities that may be suitable for clients with specific postures of the shoulder and state for which clients these self-management tools might be contraindicated.

The four postures covered in this chapter are protracted scapula, internal rotation of the humerus, winged scapula and elevated scapula. These may be related to postures described elsewhere in this book: protracted scapula and internal rotation of the humerus are associated with thoracic kyphosis (chapter 4); elevation of the scapula is often observed to coincide with a laterally flexed neck (chapter 3).

Protracted Scapula

Protraction is movement of the scapula around the rib cage. When a patient is described as having a protracted scapula, the scapula is abducted with respect to the spine and rests in a more anterior position than normal (figure 9.1).

A common method of assessing the position of the scapula is to measure the distance between the medial border of the scapula and the midline of the body (figure 9.1). When the scapula protracts, this distance increases. It is difficult to state precisely how anterior a scapula should lie for it to be termed *protracted*. It has often been cited that in the normal posture the medial border of the scapula lies approximately 2 inches (5 cm) from the midline of the body (e.g., Brunstromm 2012), perhaps because this was the figure given by Hoppenfeld (1976); but a study by Sobush and colleagues (1996) found scapular position to be greater than 3.25 inches (8.3 cm) from the spine. As with many studies, different methods give rise to different findings. Sobush and colleagues studied healthy young women, a very specific group, whereas other studies have taken measurements from an older or more varied population or from cadavers rather than living participants. We cannot even be certain that in a 'normal' posture scapulae should be approximately equidistant from the spine, because there may be variation in this also. Kendall and colleagues (1993) reported patients tended to have a lower scapula on the dominant arm, and Sobush and colleagues found the scapula of the dominant arm to be further away (more protracted or abducted) from the midline than the spine, compared to the non-dominant arm.

Another difficulty in assessing for protraction is that scapulae can rotate in a motion that is termed *rotatory winging* (Magee 2002), where the inferior angle of a scapula moves further away from the midline of the body than the superior angle. Another term for this is *upward rotation* (figure 9.2). A scapula that is upwardly rotated might therefore appear to be more protracted. In sportspeople there may be marked asymmetry in the

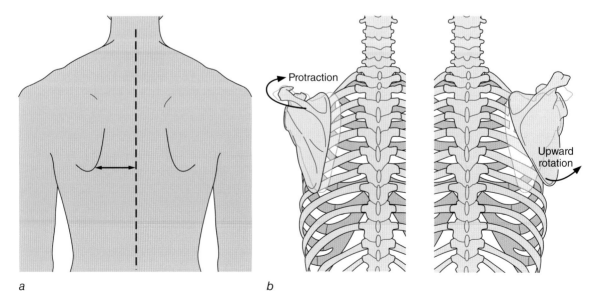

a *b*

Figure 9.1 *(a)* Normal scapular position; *(b)* protracted scapular position.

Figure 9.2 Rotatory winging (upward scapular rotation).

Consequences of Protracted Scapular Posture

In this posture soft tissues on the anterior chest and shoulder are shortened whilst those on the upper back and posterior shoulder are lengthened. The muscles responsible for holding the scapula in place are trapezius, serratus anterior, rhomboids and levator scapulae. Changes to the resting position of the scapula affect the lengths of these muscles. Long-term changes to length may weaken them and impair proper shoulder function. When neuromuscular control is altered, it results in abnormal movement patterns, which could impair sporting performance. Altering the length–tension relationship between internal rotators of the humerus and external rotators of the humerus may be one reason why scapular protraction has been significantly related to shoulder overuse injuries. However, one study found no significant difference in the resting position of the scapula between healthy patients and those with shoulder overuse injuries (Greenfield et al. 1995).

Scapular protraction is related to a narrow subacromial space, increased strain on the anterioinferior glenohumeral ligament, reduced impingement-free arc of the upper limb through elevation, reduced isometric abduction strength and reduced isometric elevation strength. A protracted scapular posture impairs rehabilitation: Restoration of shoulder rotation strength may be jeopardized if the scapula is abnormally positioned (Smith et al. 2006). The position of the humerus is affected. Attached to the scapula at the glenoid fossa, the humerus follows the movement of the scapula and it too is brought forward, falling into more internal rotation than normal. Internal rotators of the humerus may be shortened with respect to external rotators. This too can compromise shoulder function. Internal rotation of the shoulder is discussed in the next section.

Abnormal shoulder positions are commonly believed to be associated with abnormal cervical and thoracic spine positions, in particular with increased thoracic kyphosis and the forward head posture, which are described in chapters 4 and 3, respectively. However, Culham and Peat (1993) found no significant difference in scapular protraction as kyphosis increased. More research is needed in order to confirm the relationships between these postures.

Table 9.1 Muscle Lengths Associated With Protracted Scapulae

Bone	Shortened muscles	Lengthened muscles
Of the scapula	Pectoralis minor Serratus anterior Upper fibres of trapezius Subscapularis	Middle and lower fibres of trapezius Rhomboids major and minor
Of the humerus	Pectoralis major Anterior fibres of deltoid Teres major Latissimus dorsi	Posterior fibres of deltoid Teres minor Infraspinatus

Note that the infraspinatus is listed as a humeral muscle because it lengthens as the humerus becomes increasingly internally rotated with this posture and does not affect the scapula itself.

shoulders. For example, the scapula on the dominant side of asymptomatic tennis players has been found to be more protracted than the scapula on the non-dominant side, and this asymmetry may be normal for this group of sportspeople (Oyama et al. 2009).

When assessing your client, it is probably wise to focus on asymmetry rather than be too concerned over actual measurements of scapular protraction and to recognize that wide variations exist and that muscle length tests will be an essential adjunct to your assessment for this posture. In table 9.1 you can see which muscles are found to be short and which lengthened. Assessment of protracted scapula is determined not only by viewing your client from behind but also by viewing him from the side and front. In the sagittal plane the protracted scapula is described as the acromion resting at a more anterior position than normal. An anterior view might reveal that the shoulders appear more prominent with a greater concavity to the anterior of the joint than is normally apparent.

Before treatment, note that caution is needed when attempting to correct the protracted scapular posture in certain client groups:

- Clients with shoulder pathologies. Postural correction is sometimes advocated as a treatment for conditions such as subacromial impingement syndrome in the belief that helping to reposition the humerus and scapula will reduce symptoms. However, great care is needed to avoid aggravating a known condition, so it is recommended that you apply only one treatment technique at a time and to get feedback from your client before progressing with a full course of treatment.

- Clients with or at risk of having osteoporosis (e.g., elderly or anorexic clients or clients *formerly* anorexic or bulimic). This is because passive stretches performed to help lengthen soft tissues on the anterior chest and shoulder place some stress on vertebrae and are therefore potentially harmful in patients with brittle bones.

- Clients who have recently had surgery to the chest or abdomen. Passive extension of the shoulders whilst in abduction helps to lengthen anterior chest and shoulder muscles but could affect wound healing.

- Clients whose postures are protective in nature, adopted consciously or unconsciously in response to emotional sensitivity (e.g., fear, anxiety, shyness, depression). Inherent to the techniques used here is a physical opening up of the anterior of the body and can leave some clients feeling emotionally exposed.

What You Can Do as a Therapist

- Acknowledge that interventions may be limited where scapular protraction coincides with kyphosis that is the result of degenerative changes rather than the poor posture associated with slumped positions.

- Help your client to identify causal factors and correct her own posture. Any activity that encourages flexion at the shoulder with increased thoracic flexion is likely to contribute to this posture. Examples are prolonged driving with the arms outstretched, hunching over when gardening, sitting at a desk, playing computer games, doing close work such as drawing, needlepoint or illustration.

- A good starting point is to grasp the scapula whilst your client is in the side-lying position and mobilize it in all directions, assessing for restrictions in movement (figure 9.3a).

■ Passively stretch shortened tissues. A popular belief is that shortening of the pectorals contributes significantly to the posture of protracted scapulae, and these muscles can sometimes be found to be shortened when tested. An early study (Fitz 1906) of 100 cadaveric specimens found that it was not the pectorals that limited movement of the scapula; rather, it was the serratus anterior. DiVeta and colleagues (1990) found no relationship between the position of the scapula in standing patients and muscular force produced by the pectorals. There are many ways to passively stretch the pectorals, such as with the client seated (figure 4.2a) or in the supine position, perhaps with a bolster positioned lengthwise down the spine, taking care to support the head (figure 4.2b). If the bolster is too firm, it can be difficult for the client to remain resting on it comfortably because there is a tendency to roll to one side unless equal pressure is applied to both shoulders. When performing the seated chest stretch, take care not to overextend the client's spine. Concentrate on extending the client's arms rather than arching the back, but take care not to overextend the shoulder. One way to make the seated pectoral stretch more comfortable is to place a pillow behind the client. This is a useful position for the application of muscle energy technique. Serratus anterior is difficult to stretch passively because stretches performed by hooking into the medial border of the scapula in order to access the muscle also stretch rhomboids, which is counterproductive. Subscapularis, teres major and the anterior fibres of the deltoid muscle are all listed in table 9.1 because with increasing protraction of the scapula there is internal rotation of the humerus and these muscles all contribute to internal rotation. For more information about treating internal rotation of the humerus, see the next section.

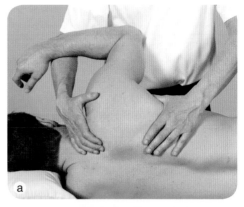

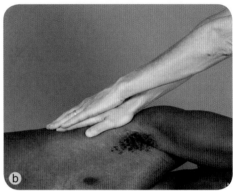

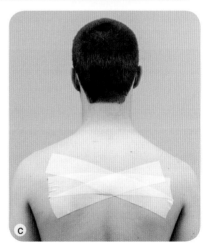

Figure 9.3 Therapist techniques for the protracted scapular posture include (a) passive scapular mobilization, (b) massage to serratus anterior and (c) taping.

■ Massage shortened tissues. The clavicular portion of the pectoral muscle can be massaged with your client supine, a position in which you have greatest leverage on these tissues (figure 4.2d). Where massage of the whole chest is acceptable, concentrate on stretching tissues from the sternum to the shoulder by using less of your massage medium than normal. Serratus anterior can best be massaged with your client in side lying (figure 9.3b), also a good position for the application of techniques such as myofascial release.

■ To enhance the stretch of chest tissues, you could use soft tissue release. Holding your client's arm so that the shoulder is flexed at about 90 degrees, gently lock the chest tissue using your fingers or first, gently pushing the tissues away from you. Maintaining your pressure, slowly abduct your client's arm, passively stretching the tissues (figure 4.2e).

■ Tape the upper back following the general taping protocol set out in chapter 2. For long-term benefit is it better to encourage your client to facilitate postural correction through strengthening of his own muscles than to encourage reliance on tape, the effects of which may be short lived. The taping pattern in figure 9.3c is an alternative to that described in the section on thoracic kyphosis based on research by Lewis and colleagues (2005). Note that evidence for the use of taping is inconclusive and there are as yet no guidelines on which client group might benefit. It may be specific to a sport or activity specific or to a patient. For example, one study found that taping to correct scapular protraction in violin players negatively affected comfort and concentration and did not enhance scapula-stabilizing muscles when applied to professional violinists (Ackermann et al. 2002).

■ Teach your client exercises such as the dart and prone rhomboid retraction to help strengthen the middle and lower fibres of trapezius and thus help retract the scapula (see chapter 4). DiVeta (1990) found no relationship between the position of the scapula and muscular force produced by the middle portion of trapezius. However, Greenfield and colleagues (1995) observe that weakness of the rhomboids and middle fibres of trapezius became more apparent as patients abducted their arms so suggest that a dysfunctional state of muscle weakness resulting in excessive scapular protraction during movement may not be apparent when a patient is assessed with arms resting at the sides in standing. The ability of the shoulder to generate isometric rotation strength is dependent on scapular position (Smith et al. 2006). Therefore, there is some justification for using manual therapy to facilitate a more normal scapular position where possible.

■ Refer your client to a professional able to provide joint mobilization. Tightness of the posterior shoulder capsule has been found to correlate with the protracted scapular posture, so stretching the capsule using joint mobilization can be beneficial.

■ Address alterations to the position of other upper-body parts that are associated with this posture (in this case forward head posture, thoracic kyphosis and internal rotation of the humerus) using the suggestions put forward in the relevant sections of this book. Note that Culham and Peat (1993) found no significant increase in the distance between the spine and scapula as kyphosis increased, as has popularly been believed.

What Your Client Can Do

■ Identify any factors that might contribute to the maintenance of protracted scapulae and avoid these where possible. Not all of the contributing factors may be avoidable (e.g., where there is an associated kyphotic posture due to degenerative changes in vertebrae). Activities that encourage flexion at the shoulder combined with a slumped posture are likely to contribute to this posture and include prolonged driving with the arms outstretched, hunching over when gardening, sitting at a desk and playing computer games.

- Strengthen the middle and lower fibres of trapezius and the rhomboid muscles to help retract scapulae using exercises such as the dart and prone rhomboid retraction (figure 4.4a). Aim to build up the time the position can be held in each exercise pose.

- Use prone rhomboid retraction by asking your client to abduct the arms to about 90 degrees and then to gently lift them off the floor and supinate the forearm so that the thumbs are pointing upwards.

- Another exercise is for your client to stand against a wall and to try to keep the shoulder blades against the wall while slowly abducting the arms and then lowering them, as if making sand or snow angels.

- Consider referral to an exercise professional for specific strengthening exercises of the middle and lower fibres of trapezius in addition to those outlined here. For example, high muscular activity in the lower fibres of trapezius occurs in prone rowing and when externally rotating the arm at 90 degrees of abduction (Escamilla et al. 2009). Specialised exercise professionals are likely to be able to design a programme to address weakened muscles where these are identified. Such a programme is likely to begin with standing, low-load activation exercises with the arm below shoulder level in order to help the client learn how to engage scapular retractor muscles (Kibler et al. 2013). Where there is imbalance in the scapular muscles, it is important for the client to learn how to activate the middle and lower fibres of the trapezius without activating the upper fibres of the muscle. Investigation into 12 exercises commonly used in rehabilitation of the shoulder girdle found side-lying external shoulder rotation, side-lying forward flexion of the shoulder, prone horizontal abduction with external rotation and prone extension to promote middle- and lower-trapezial activity with minimal activation of the upper trapezius (Cools et al. 2007). However, the authors acknowledge that functional activity is superior to static exercises such as those described but note that it is very difficult to modify these exercises so that they resemble daily activities or sport-specific functions.

- Actively stretch shortened muscles, in this case the pectorals and serratus anterior. Stretch the internal shoulder rotators, subscapularis, teres major and anterior fibres of the deltoid where these are found to be shortened. Contraction of the rhomboids is a simple method of lengthening the soft tissues on the anterior chest wall and can be performed surreptitiously almost anywhere (figure 4.4a). Actively stretching pectorals can be performed in standing using a towel (figure 4.4c) or wall for assistance or resting in the supine position over a bolster (figure 4.4b).

- When using a wall or doorframe to facilitate a chest stretch, encourage your client to experiment with placing the arm at various degrees of abduction or elevation and then turn the body away from the wall. Different arm positions localise the stretch to different regions of the chest, and in this manner the client can learn to identify areas of tension.

- Use a foam roller to facilitate spinal extension (figure 4.4d). Use extreme care because these rollers are made of firm Styrofoam as used in this manner and place considerable pressure on individual vertebrae. Use of these rollers would be contraindicated for anyone with osteoporosis or a history of thoracic spinal pathology (such as joint subluxation or disc herniation), and clients with inflammatory conditions such as rheumatoid arthritis should use them cautiously.

- Consider using a shoulder brace for short periods. Braces provide the client with an opportunity to experience a more normal scapular position. However, they should only be used for short periods. Active strengthening of weak muscles is preferable for helping to regain a more normal scapular position rather than relying on a mechanical aid to retain good posture. Braces have been found to improve scapular posture, but their effect on muscle activation is highly variable (Cole et al. 2013).

- Address any forward head posture or internal rotation of the humerus using the suggestions in the relevant sections in this book.

Internal Rotation of the Humerus

The humerus rests in slight internal rotation in the normal posture (figure 9.4a) but in some patients may be exaggerated. Internal rotation coincides with scapular protraction so may be more prevalent in patients whose scapulae are more protracted than normal. When a patient has a more pronounced internal rotation of the arm than normal, internal rotator muscles are shortened and muscle length tests are used to confirm this. However, when observing your client from behind, the position of the elbow provides a clue to this posture because the olecranon rotates away from you, as in the case of the patient's left arm in figure 9.4b. Observation of the hand can also be useful as more of the palm becomes visible with increasing internal rotation of the shoulder. Note that a more visible hand does not guarantee your client has an internally rotated shoulder. Increased visibility of the palm can also be the result of increased supination in the forearm.

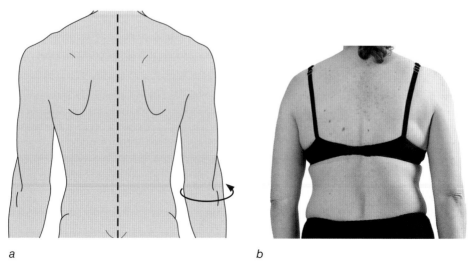

a   b

Figure 9.4 Normal shoulder posture and elbow position (a), and (b) exaggerated internal rotation of the humerus.

Consequences of Internal Rotation of the Humerus

The main consequence of this posture is the increased likelihood of developing a shoulder impingement condition. In the normal shoulder posture, the humeral head hangs in the glenoid fossa (figure 9.5) and the arm may be flexed quite comfortably to 90 degrees and right up into elevation. However, as the head of the humerus rotates around its longitudinal axis (usually with scapular protraction), the greater tubercle rests more anteriorly compared to normal, and on elevation of the arm is more likely to compress soft tissues beneath the acromion, causing pain and limiting movement.

You can see in table 9.2 that internal rotators are shortened and are likely to be weakened, and external rotators are lengthened and also likely to be weakened. Weakness in infraspinatus and teres minor reduces the ability of the rotator cuff to control upward shear of the humeral head when the deltoid muscle contracts during abduction of the arm. This could account for the increased likelihood of impingement of the humeral head in the subacromial space. On a daily basis, patients with this condition may have pain on certain movements and a reduced ability to externally rotate the arm. Individuals can tolerate this posture for many months or even years before suddenly feeling pain, because muscular adaptation evolves over time until the point at which movement results in impingement. This posture is associated with protracted shoulders and a forward head position. Tables 3.3 and 9.1 detail muscle imbalances associated with these two respective postures.

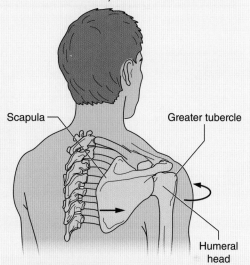

Scapula

Greater tubercle

Humeral head

Figure 9.5 Change in humeral and scapular positions when a patient has an internally rotated humerus. Arrows indicate position change for an internally rotated humerus with corresponding protraction of the scapula.

Table 9.2 Muscle Lengths Associated With Internal Rotation of the Humerus

Area	Shortened muscles	Lengthened muscles
Superficial	Pectoralis major Anterior fibers of deltoid Latissimus dorsi	Infraspinatus Posterior fibres of deltoid
Deep	Teres major Pectoralis minor	Teres minor Supraspinatus

What You Can Do as a Therapist

Use caution when attempting to correct internal rotation of the humerus in certain clients. These include clients prone to subluxations or dislocations of the shoulder, those with known hypermobility syndromes, those with arthritis in the shoulder or clients you suspect have adhesive capsulitis. Overstretching could aggravate these conditions.

- Help your client to identify factors that may contribute to this posture, such as sitting with protracted scapulae or repetitively performing movements that demand internal rotation of the shoulder, as may be the case in certain manual occupations.

- Teach your client how to stretch the internal rotators of the humerus and strengthen the external rotators. Self-correction of posture is always preferable to therapeutic intervention where this is possible.

- Passively stretch shortened tissues. Where internal rotation has caused acute symptoms, approach correction of the posture with caution so as to avoid a flare-up of symptoms. A good starting point is to gently traction the joint (figure 9.6a), taking care to grasp the arm above the elbow to avoid also tractioning the elbow. This has

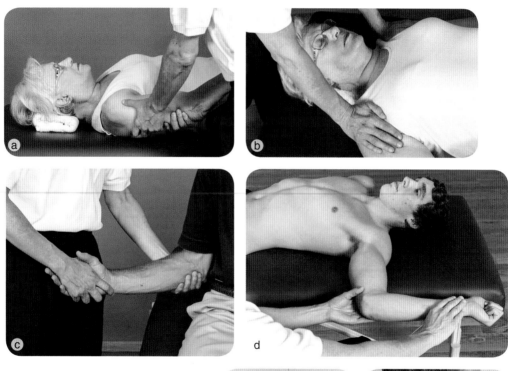

Figure 9.6 Therapist techniques for internal rotation of the humerus include (a) gentle traction of the glenohumeral joint, (b) gentle compression of the shoulders and (b) passive stretch in (c) seated and (d) supine positions plus taping using patterns designed to encourage (e) external rotation and (f) correct scapular position.

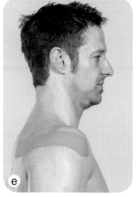
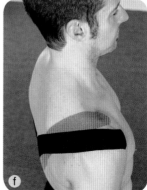

the effect of stretching tissues of the joint as a group before more specific stretches. Placing your hands bilaterally on the shoulders and applying gentle compression (figure 9.6b) stretches anterior shoulder tissues and gently moves the humeral head posteriorly in the joint. This too is a good initial stretch, more tolerable than attempting to take the arm into external rotation. With your client seated, you could attempt gentle lateral rotation, supporting your client's elbow (figure 9.6c). One of the disadvantages to this technique is that it is difficult to apply gentle overpressure without the client rotating the trunk towards you. It does, however, enable your client to keep the arm adducted if that is more comfortable. This can then progress to passive lateral rotation with the client supine (figure 9.6d). Note that where internal rotation is marked, the client is usually unable to abduct or externally rotate the arm to the degree shown in figure 9.6d. Either seated or supine positions can be used to apply muscle energy technique.

- Massage shortened muscles, in this case the internal rotators of the humerus, where these are accessible. The pectoralis major and anterior deltoid are obvious choices for massage (figure 4.2d). You could also palpate and address tension in teres major and latissimus dorsi on the lateral border of the scapula with your client in a prone or side-lying position.

- Apply tape. Ask your client to sit up straight and to gently retract and depress the scapula to achieve a more normal position. If possible, help position your client's arm so that it is not internally rotated. Apply tape to encourage lateral rotation of the humerus (figure 9.6e) and to discourage scapular protraction (figure 9.6f). Any tape used must not restrict movement but provide proprioceptive feedback to the client to help avoid positions of scapular protraction and internal rotation of the shoulder. It is always preferable for a client to learn to strengthen weak muscles in an attempt to correct posture rather than to rely on the use of tape.

- Treat for forward head posture and protracted scapulae where these are present by using the suggestions in the relevant sections of this book.

What Your Client Can Do

- Identify and avoid factors that may contribute to this posture, such as sitting with protracted scapulae or repetitively performing movements that demand internal rotation of the shoulder.

- Rest in positions that encourage passive lengthening of the internal rotators of the shoulder. This could mean resting supine as if about to receive a passive stretch, shown in figure 9.6d, or you could teach your client how to use pillows on which to rest the hand if sitting is preferable (figure 9.7a).

- Actively stretch internal rotators of the shoulder. There are various ways to do this, one of which is to stand in a doorway and use the frame for resistance (figure 9.7b).

- Strengthen external rotators of the shoulder. This can be achieved by using a resistance band with the shoulder adducted (figure 9.7c) or abducted (figure 9.7d). It is important for your client to start the exercise with the scapula in a good position, gently retracted and depressed rather than protracted. A useful but more challenging method is for the client to try to stretch a resistance band by using both arms, which encourages activation of the external rotator muscles, then to maintain this position whilst raising and lowering the arms (figure 9.7e).

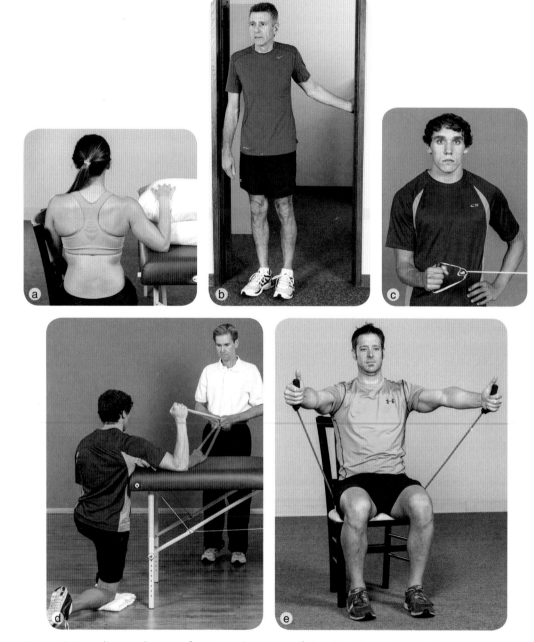

Figure 9.7 Client techniques for internal rotation of the shoulder include *(a)* resting in positions that encourage passive stretch of internal rotator muscles, *(b)* active stretch of internal rotators, strengthening of external shoulder rotators unilaterally with the arm *(c)* adducted or *(d)* abducted or *(e)* bilaterally using a resistance band.

Winged Scapula

In asymptomatic patients the scapula rests approximately 10 to 20 degrees from the spine, or vertical plane (Levangie and Norkin 2001) and has the ability to tilt in the sagittal plane (figure 9.8). Also called scapula alata, scapular winging is a condition in which the inferior angle and medial border of the scapula protrude in a prominent manner from the thorax (Tibaek and Gadsboell 2014). There are varying degrees of normal scapular tilt. For example, one study found that scapular tilt increased with age and averaged 13.2 degrees in women over age 50 (Culham and Peat 1993). However, there is no mistaking the appearance of a winged scapula, which is prominent and usually markedly asymmetrical. Winging is usually evident when the patient stands with the arm by the side and the medial and inferior borders of the scapula are observed to be closer to the spine and lifted superiorly compared to the unaffected side and is accentuated when the client flexes the shoulder forward to a horizontal position (Martin and Fish 2008). This posture is usually due to damage to the long thoracic nerve, which serves the serratus anterior. Serratus anterior, therefore, no longer acts to hold the scapula against the chest wall. In

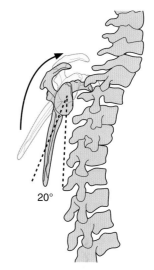

Figure 9.8 Normal scapular position and tilt and winged scapula.

Consequences of Scapular Winging

Scapular winging has been cited as one of the factors attributed to overuse injuries (Greenfield et al. 1995). This could be because scapular tilt decreases the subacromial space and therefore increases the risk of soft tissue impingement (Escamilla et al. 2009). However, it is not always clear whether the term *scapular tilt* refers to tilt that is within normal parameters, or whether the term *winging* has been used to mean scapular tilt rather than true scapular winging. True winging affects the entire shoulder girdle. There is often pain in the neck, shoulder and upper back (Meininger et al. 2011) with patients concerned about appearance (Klebe et al. 2003). Without stability of the scapula, people with this condition have difficulty elevating the arm overhead and may rely on upper fibres of the trapezius and lateral flexion of the trunk as a compensatory mechanism. There is difficulty with everyday tasks such as pushing open a door.

Table 9.3   Muscle Changes Associated With Winged Scapula

Area	Effect on joints	Length–tension effects
Paralysis of serratus anterior muscle	Scapula is no longer held against chest wall Abnormal scapulothoracic function Abnormal glenohumeral joint function	Tight or shortened pectoralis minor; where protraction is also present, shortening of internal rotators of the humerus

some cases injury to the spinal accessory nerve results in paralysis of the upper trapezius and, in this case, causes winging of the lateral border. In athletes the medial border may be more prominent perhaps because of tightness in pectoralis minor (Forthomme et al. 2008), but this is not scapular winging.

What You Can Do as a Therapist

Unfortunately there is little that can be done by using massage and stretching techniques for this posture. In some cases the condition resolves over time, but injury to the long thoracic nerve or to the spinal accessory nerve can take 6 months to 2 years to heal (Cabrera et al. 2014). Bracing has been found to be effective (Klebe et al. 2003). Early braces were a simple strap apparatus designed to keep a pad fixed over the scapula. Modern braces are designed to achieve the same function but are made of more lightweight, often washable materials.

- Maintaining range of motion in the shoulder is important in preventing contracture of pericapsular soft tissues, but take care not to overstretch the paralyzed muscle (Martin and Fish 2008). Maintaining range of motion (ROM) could be achieved with gentle passive mobilization of the shoulder or by teaching your client how to rest in a posture that facilitates relaxation in various ranges within each movement. This is preferable to active ROM exercises, which would necessitate the use of muscles in such a way that might exacerbate the existing muscular imbalance.

- Where therapy can help is in identifying shortened muscles or those that feel palpably tight and using massage or stretching to facilitate lengthening. Pectoralis minor may be particularly tight, as are all of the soft tissues around the anterior of the shoulder.

- Refer to a specialist physiotherapist for rehabilitative exercise. Strengthening exercises should be started only once reinnervation of the affected muscle has been confirmed (Martin and Fish 2008). Where the condition does not resolve, surgery is used plus a programme of physiotherapy in which these specialized exercises (termed scaption exercises) are tailored to individual patients. Tibaek and Gadsboell (2014) describe a rehabilitation programme that includes exercises such as passive positioning of the scapula in an upwardly rotated position in either the prone (figure 9.9a) or supine positions to facilitate mobilization and general capsular stretch. Another exercise is to retract the scapula whilst in the supine position (figure 9.9b). A third, more difficult, exercise is to rest supine in order to keep the scapula in place against the floor and to slowly stretch a rubber tube or band from a vertical position up into elevation and return to vertical, using the other hand as an anchor for the tube or band (figure 9.9c). Scaption exercises also focus on helping the client to regain control of specific muscles, in this case by giving the client instructions to make the arm longer (figure 9.9d) or shorter (figure 9.9e). It is important to note that these are highly specialized exercises and should be performed under guidance initially in order to determine the correct number of sets and repetitions and whether the client is performing the exercise correctly.

What Your Client Can Do

Follow the exercise advice given by a physiotherapist or exercise professional. Exercises focus on gaining control of the lower fibres of the trapezius and, eventually, in serratus anterior where this is possible.

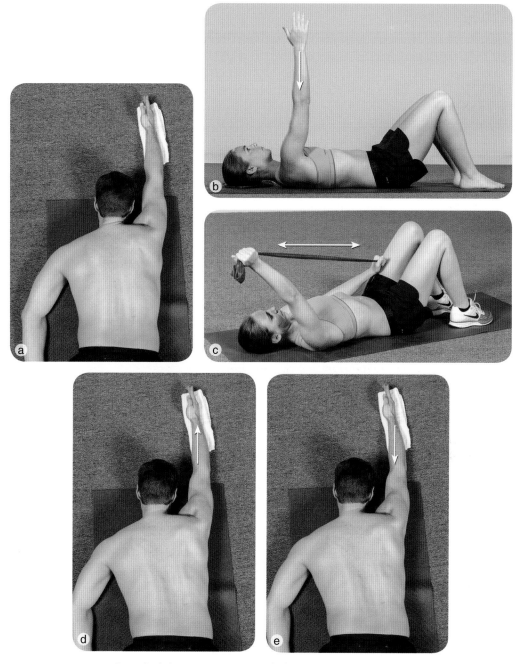

Figure 9.9 Specialist rehabilitation exercise include passive positioning of the scapula in (a) upward rotation, (b) supine scapular protraction or retraction, (c) resistance exercise focusing on control of lower fibres of trapezius, scaption exercises where the client is instructed to make the arm (d) longer or (e) shorter.

Elevated Shoulder

The scapula usually rests over ribs 2 to 7 between thoracic levels T2 and T7 (Brunstromm 2012). When it is drawn upwards it is said to be elevated; the opposite is when it rests lower and is said to be depressed, both of which are normal scapular movements (figure 9.10a). In some patients the scapula remains elevated, as can be seen in the right shoulder in figure 9.10b. The scapula of the non-dominant arm is often lower than the dominant arm (Kendall et al. 1993). In overhead athletes the dominant shoulder is often positioned lower than the non-dominant shoulder, perhaps due to stretching of ligaments and joint capsules repetitively in a forceful manner (Oyama et al. 2008). Note that the posture described here is different to Sprengel deformity, which is a congenital condition resulting from an undescended scapula.

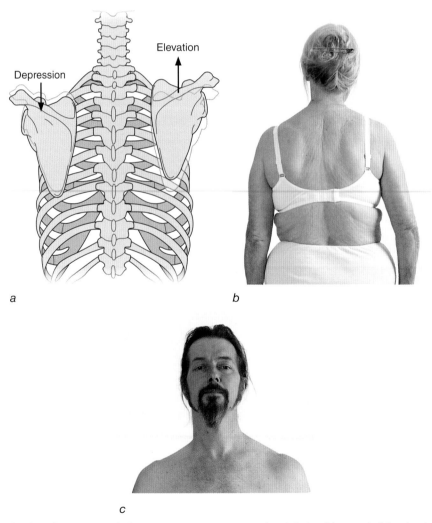

Figure 9.10 Elevation and depression movements in the (a) shoulder and (b) right shoulder elevation. (c) Elevation of the left shoulder showing asymmetry in upper trapezius.

Consequences of Elevated Shoulder

The muscles responsible for holding the scapula in place are trapezius, serratus anterior, rhomboids and levator scapulae. Changes to the resting position of the scapula affect the lengths of these muscles. Long-term changes to their length may weaken them and impair proper shoulder function. The shoulder may appear higher anteriorly (figure 9.10c) as well as posteriorly, and there could even be hypertrophy of the elevators.

Soft tissues of the neck on the side of the elevated shoulder are compressed slightly, and those on the opposite side of the neck are lengthened. Because scapular elevators also attach to the neck, if prolonged, this posture could adversely affect neck function.

Table 9.4   Muscle Lengths Associated With Elevated Shoulder

Area	Shortened muscles	Lengthened muscles
Shoulder	Upper trapezius Levator scapulae	Serratus anterior Lower trapezius

What You Can Do as a Therapist

- Help your client to identify the sorts of activities that could contribute to this posture. Examples include carrying a heavy bag on one shoulder, resting the arm (on the raised side) on the window sill of a vehicle while driving, repetitive motion of the arm above 90 degrees abduction (as in racquet sports) and wearing an arm sling that is too short.

- Help your client to compare how the left and right shoulders feel when gently depressed and thus identify any imbalance. A simple instruction is to ask the client to sit up straight with elbows relaxed at about 90 degrees of flexion and to press the elbows to the floor.

- Help your client to strengthen muscles of depression. This time, instead of pressing the elbows to the floor, ask your client to press the elbows into the armrests of a chair.

- Passively depress the shoulder. There are two simple ways to do this. One way is to ask your client to adopt normal sitting posture and to relax the shoulders. Holding the arm, gently depress the shoulder. The other method is performed with your client in the supine position (figure 9.11).

- Passively stretch levator scapulae and trapezius. With your client resting with the head in a neutral

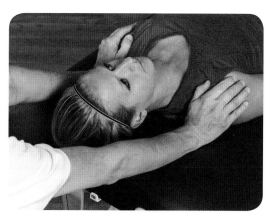

Figure 9.11   Therapist techniques for an elevated scapula include passive depression of the scapula in the supine position.

position, apply very slight traction, taking care to place your hands superior to the elbow joint. As you maintain this traction, ask your client to slowly perform lateral flexion away from you (figure 3.5a). In this illustration the patient is being treated for elevation of the right scapula. Obviously this tractions the glenohumeral joint so is contraindicated for clients with dislocating or subluxing shoulders and must be performed with care on clients who are hypermobile. Or you could apply gentle overpressure to either the shoulder or the head or both, in either sitting or supine position (figure 3.5b).

- Massage shortened tissues, in this case the upper fibres of the trapezius and levator scapulae.

- Apply soft tissue release on the elevated side (figure 3.5c).

- Teach your client how to stretch the muscles on the side of the neck to which it is flexed.

What Your Client Can Do

- Identify and avoid activities that contribute to prolonged elevation of the scapula.

- Practice scapular depression exercises. These have the advantage of strengthening muscles of depression whilst inhibiting those of elevation. Whilst seated, the client presses the elbows into the arms of the chair or, keeping the elbows extended, tries to lift himself upwards (figure 9.12).

- Actively stretch shortened muscles. These will be on the side of the neck of the affected shoulder. Applying gentle overpressure with one hand enhances this stretch (figure 3.6a). Taking the arm behind the body is a variation on this stretch (figure 3.6b).

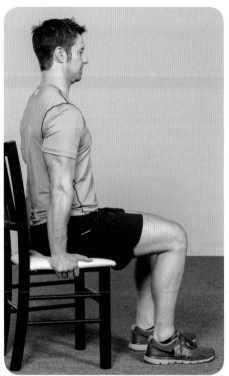

Figure 9.12 Client techniques for an elevated shoulder include scapular depression exercises.

Closing Remarks

In this chapter you learnt about four common shoulder postures: protracted scapula, internal rotation of the humerus, winged scapula and elevated shoulder. The anatomical features of each are described along with photographic examples and illustrations. The consequences of each posture are presented, and for each pathology a table is provided with lists of shortened and lengthened muscles that may help you plan your treatments.

Elbow

Learning Outcomes

After reading this chapter, you should be able to do the following:

- Describe two postures common to the elbow.
- Recognize the described postures on a client.
- Give examples of the anatomical consequences of each posture.
- Name the muscles that are shortened and those that are lengthened in each posture.
- Give examples of appropriate treatments for the correction of each posture.
- Give the rationale for such treatments and state for which clients a particular treatment is contraindicated and why.
- Give examples of the kinds of stretches, exercises and activities that may be suitable for clients with specific postures of the elbow and state for which clients these self-management tools might be contraindicated.

The two postures in this chapter are flexed elbow and hyperextended elbow. The first is often due to injury or, in some cases, overtraining of the elbow flexors; the second is due to laxity in the joint. Neither is common in the general population, but both are included because correct elbow alignment is important for proper functioning of the upper limb.

Flexed Elbow

People with flexed elbow posture stand with their elbows resting at a greater degree of flexion than normal. This is apparent when viewing your client both laterally and posteriorly (figure 10.1a and b). The resting position of a normal elbow joint is frequently cited as 70 degrees of flexion with 10 degrees of forearm supination (Magee 2002) (figure 10.2a). However, there is a wide variety of resting positions of the elbow (figure 10.2), none of which replicates this level of flexion as a resting posture. Furthermore, patients who are unable to extend their elbows, that is to have a noticeably flexed elbow posture at rest, demonstrate resting postures of *less than* 70 degrees, not more (figure 10.2). However, these patients are asymptomatic, examples of the kinds of elbow postures you may come across in general practice. Note that the patient in figure 10.2 is holding her right hand against her thigh (and increasing the elevation of her right shoulder) and may exhibit a greater degree of flexion if she were to stand without fixing her hand.

There are many reasons why you might observe a client stand with a greater degree of elbow flexion, the most common being that the elbow is stiff. A stiff elbow has been defined as loss of extension of greater than 30 degrees and flexion of less than 120 degrees (Nandi et al. 2009) (figure 10.2a). Bone and soft tissues form mechanical blocks to elbow extension and occur for a variety of reasons. For example, prolonged

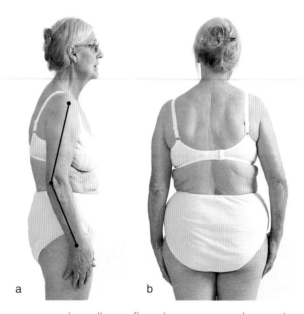

a   b

Figure 10.1 When a patient has elbows flexed to a greater degree than normal, this can be observed *(a)* laterally and *(b)* posteriorly.

immobilization of the elbow in 90 degrees of flexion results in adaptive shortening of the elbow flexors and lengthening of the elbow extensors (Levangie and Norkin 2001), intra-articular elbow pathology is often followed by contracture of the articular capsule and collateral ligaments as well as the muscles (Nandi 2009), and burns may result in loss of skin extensibility. People engaged in sports that require excessive training of elbow flexors are sometimes observed to stand with a greater degree of flexion than normal as the result of training-induced shortening of elbow flexors. Elbow extension may be limited and bony impingement may result from trauma or surgery. Extension may also be limited in patients with arthritis as a result of changes to the articular surfaces of the joint. Contraction of elbow flexors is also reported after head trauma.

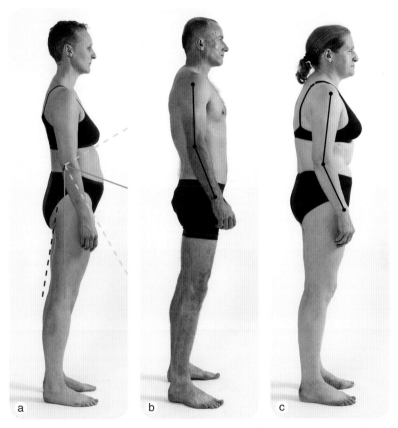

Figure 10.2 Variations in normal resting posture of the elbow. These examples demonstrate a range from about (a) 5 degrees to (b) 45 degrees (c). Some sources cite the normal resting posture of the elbow at 70 degrees of flexion, which would be the angle presented by the bold line in figure 10.2a.

Consequences of Flexed Elbow Posture

Most of the activities of daily living—such as washing, dressing, cooking and cleaning—can be performed with elbow flexion ranging from 30 to 130 degrees (Morrey et al. 1981). So unless the elbow is permanently fixed in *one* position, this posture does not affect much of daily life. However, to achieve normal function, a patient may employ compensatory movement with the shoulder and wrist, which could lead to the development of problems in those joints and with the muscles associated with them.

One of the consequences of a reduced ability to extend the elbow is that it also affects supination and pronation. A patient may be hindered in specific tasks that require these motions (e.g., turning a key in a lock or using a screwdriver).

The inability to fully extend the elbow considerably affects weight bearing. In this posture, transferring weight through a flexed joint is less stable than weight bearing through an extended joint and places greater strain on muscles and ligaments.

This posture could be limiting during exercise or sports. For example, an inability to fully extend would impair performance in racquet sports and in weight training activities such as push-ups and chest and shoulder press. If such activities were to be sustained, this could increase the likelihood of damage to the joint.

Table 10.1 Muscle Lengths Associated With Flexed Elbow

Area	Shortened muscles	Lengthened muscles
Primary muscles	Brachialis Biceps brachii Brachioradialis	Triceps brachii Anconeus
Secondary muscles	Pronator teres Flexor carpi radialis Flexor carpi ulnaris Flexor digitorum superficialis Palmaris longus	N/a

TIP Extension is also limited by the medial collateral ligament and the skin and fascia on the anterior surface of the upper limb.

What You Can Do as a Therapist

Whether you can treat a client effectively with a flexed elbow depends entirely on the aetiology of the condition affecting your client. Stiffness in the joint is a common symptom after surgery to the elbow. In this case, lengthening of the soft tissue of the anterior compartment of the elbow and strengthening of the posterior compartment, combined with mobilization of the joint, could be viable treatment suggestions. However, stiff elbows resulting from burns or from muscle contraction due to head injury are less treatable with hands-on therapy. That is not to say that hands-on therapy would not provide other valuable benefits, only that it will be less effective in changing posture of the joint. Caution is needed when treating clients with flexed elbows resulting from arthritis in the joint. Where extension is limited by bony impingement, hands-on therapy is ineffective.

- Apply passive stretches to the elbow flexors. This could involve focusing on the elbow initially (figure 10.3*a*) and then progressing to stretching wrist flexors (figure 10.3*b*). Remember to include an assessment of pronation and supination and apply passive stretches where you identify restriction. A good handhold for encouraging pronation and supination is shown in figure 10.3*c*. Higher-intensity, prolonged, and frequent stretching may be beneficial for certain hypomobility problems when used as an adjunct to high-grade mobilizations (Jacobs and Sciascia 2011). Static stretching three times for 30 minutes daily has been advocated for post-traumatic and postsurgical elbow stiffness where the stiffness is due to soft tissue rather than osseous restriction (Müller et al. 2013). Chronic contractures are less responsive to stretching, and there may be smaller improvements in range of motion (Jacobs and Sciascia 2011).

- Referral to a physiotherapist or osteopath who could provide joint mobilizations if these are not something that falls within your remit. Physiotherapeutic treatment for fixed-flexion contracture of the elbow is varied. One study showed that use of a low-load, prolonged stretch applied via a splint increased the range of motion for

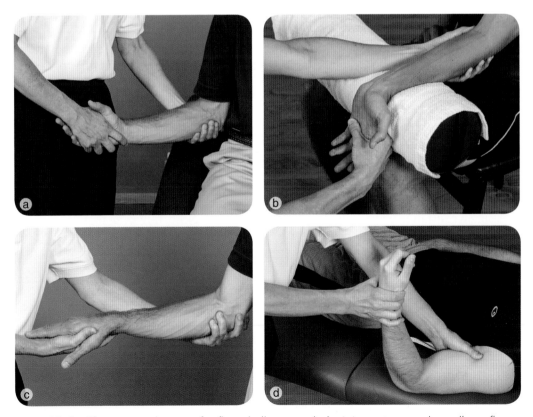

Figure 10.3 Therapist techniques for flexed elbows include *(a)* passive stretch to elbow flexors without wrist flexors, *(b)* building up to incorporate stretches to wrist flexors, *(c)* using stretches to encourage supination and pronation and *(d)* using techniques such as soft tissue release.

elbow flexion contracture where this was due to neurologic aetiology after head trauma (MacKay-Lyons 1989).

- Massage the elbow flexors in order to lengthen them. This could involve simple stripping type strokes to the arm or involve soft tissue release technique where a point on the arm is fixed (figure 10.3d) and then the elbow extended whilst retaining pressure on the fixed point. One of the advantages of using soft tissue release to encourage elbow extension is that you do not need to take the elbow beyond its current extension range in order to stretch the elbow flexors. Soft tissue release is also beneficial for lengthening the wrist flexors and could be used similarly.

- Refer your client to a practitioner who is able to provide splinting. Where moderate loss of extension is due to soft tissue contractures, a dynamic splint has been found to be effective, but there is a time limit during which this may be used effectively (Nandi 2009).

- Teach your client how to stretch elbow flexor muscles.

What Your Client Can Do

- Rest in positions that encourage elbow extension. A client with a flexed elbow (figure 10.4a) could rest with the elbow on a cushion and use the weight of the hand and forearm to gently stretch the soft tissues of the anterior elbow.

- Perform active stretches for the elbow flexors. The most effective method is to grasp a doorframe or pole with the shoulder internally rotated and the elbow extended and forearm pronated, the thumb pointing downward (Alter 2004). This could be a difficult position for some clients to adopt. A simple start is for your client to use the hand of the other arm to encourage extension of the joint on a daily basis (figure 10.4b). Stretches to the wrist flexors are useful because these muscles cross the elbow joint on the anterior surface and lengthening them could facilitate extension (10.4c).

- Practice contracting the triceps, which encourages relaxation of main elbow flexors through the mechanism of reciprocal inhibition and could be valuable in lengthening elbow flexors. Triceps weaken if lengthened, and practicing non-weight-bearing triceps strengthening exercise is likely to be beneficial in correcting a flexed elbow posture where this is due to soft tissue shortening alone. One way to do this is by using a resistance band whilst seated (figure 10.4d). Note, however, that the motion of gripping uses wrist and finger flexors, most of which cross the anterior elbow joint and contribute to elbow flexion, so gripping should be minimized.

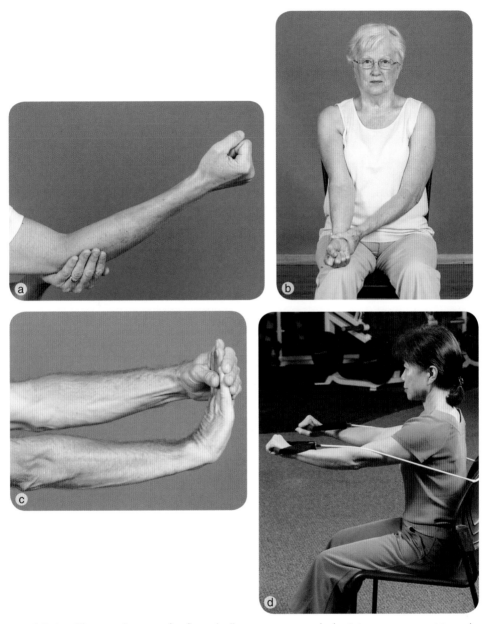

Figure 10.4 Client techniques for flexed elbow posture include *(a)* resting in positions that encourage elbow extension, *(b)* using the other hand to facilitate stretch of elbow flexors, *(c)* stretching wrist flexors and *(d)* performing non-weight-bearing exercises to strengthen triceps.

Hyperextended Elbow

In adults, there is minimal, if any, elbow extension; where this is present it is around 0 to 10 degrees (American Academy of Orthopaedic Surgeons 1994). Extension greater than 10 degrees is considered hyperextension. This posture is not easy to spot when a person is standing with arms relaxed. It becomes apparent when the person performs active elbow extension and the end of range position is observed to be greater than normal.

Consequences of Hyperextended Elbow

In this posture the soft tissues on the anterior of the arm are lengthened and those on the posterior of the arm are shortened. During activities requiring resistance or weight bearing there is reduced stability in the joint and greater risk of injury to soft tissues. Where the joint is forced further into extension, there may be injury to the olecranon fossa as the olecranon is forced into it. There is sometimes pain in the joint or in other joints of the upper limb as extra strain is placed on shoulders and wrists as a result of altered biomechanics. Where the posture is the result of hypermobility syndrome, there is likely to be a range of musculoskeletal (Kirk et al. 1967) and non-musculoskeletal symptoms, including proprioceptive deficit (Kaux et al. 2013). There is risk of injury to the elbow during sporting activity, and hyperextension could impair performance.

Table 10.2 Muscle Lengths Associated With Hyperextended Elbow

Area	Shortened muscles	Lengthened muscles
Arm	Triceps Anconeus	Biceps brachii Brachialis Brachioradialis
Forearm	Elbow extensors	Elbow flexors

TIP When a patient has one of the hypermobility syndromes, she has greater extensibility in the soft tissues of joints throughout the body, not just at the elbow. The categorization of muscles in table 10.2 may not apply for this group of patients who may have extensibility in both flexors and extensors of the elbow and no shortened muscles at all.

What You Can Do as a Therapist

Note that specialist advice is needed when working with clients with known hypermobility syndromes because these clients are at risk of injury from both stretching and strengthening programmes that must be supervised initially to ensure correct technique.

- With this posture the most important treatment is to advise your client on self-correction. Teach your client what a neutral (0-degree) position is for elbow extension and help the client identify times when he may take the elbow beyond this position (e.g., resting on the hands when the hands are behind the back when seated; levering oneself out from the side of a swimming pool; leaning through one hand when kneeling to wash a floor, play with young children, or exercise). Demonstrate correct elbow alignment, especially during weight-bearing activities.

- Teach the client to avoid hyperextension of the joint and practice first in non-weight-bearing activities, then during resistance exercise, and finally during simple weight bearing.

- Advise your client on suitable strengthening exercises for the elbow flexor muscles. If necessary, refer your client to a fitness professional who will provide exercises for elbow flexors in a way that avoids hyperextension of the elbow. Eccentric exercises using an isokinetic device may be used to train muscles so that these act as a protective break to joint hypermobility (Kaux et al. 2013). A fitness professional may also advise on how to avoid hyperextension when performing regular strength training activities such as push-up, chest press, shoulder press, and triceps extension.

- Consider taping the elbow. Taping can physically prevent hyperextension or can be applied so that hyperextension is possible, but in doing so the tape is tensioned, providing sensory feedback to the client who can then self-correct the position of the elbow and eventually learn not to extend beyond around 0 degrees. The tape pattern you use could be as simple as a strip placed lengthwise over the elbow (figure 10.5a) or in a cross shape (figure 10.5b).

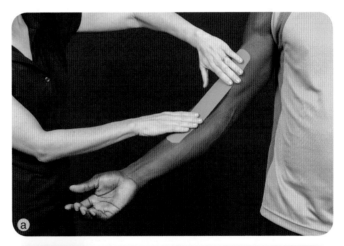

- Massage triceps only of this is found to be shortened but not if your client has a known hypermobility syndrome. Massage wrist extensors if these are found to be shortened.

- Advise your client about correct stretching technique but not if your client has a known hypermobility syndrome. If triceps and wrist extensors are found to be shortened, demonstrate safe stretches.

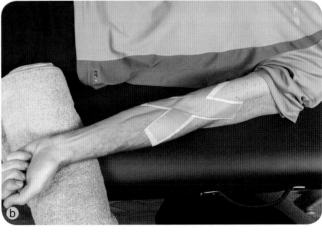

Figure 10.5 Therapist techniques for hyperextending elbows include taping using a (a) simple longitudinal strip or (b) a cross shape.

What Your Client Can Do

- Identify and modify activities where hyperextension of the elbow is encouraged. For example, when sleeping, avoid resting on the back with the arm over a pillow or edge of the bed. Learn how to bear weight through the elbow joint safely. Instead of hyperextending the elbows, practice weight bearing through a neutral elbow (figure 10.6).

- Strengthen elbow flexors using exercises such as simple biceps curls. When using weights to perform biceps curls, correcting upper-limb alignment is essential, so follow the advice provided by a fitness instructor or physiotherapist. Exercises that involve long-lever movements are potentially damaging for clients with hyperextending elbows, so care is needed in both selecting and performing exercises using weights or other forms of resistance.

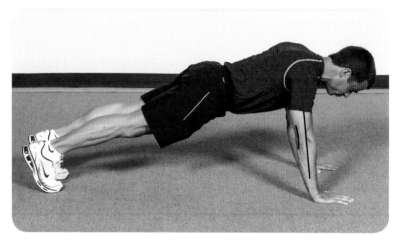

Figure 10.6 Client techniques for hyperextending elbows include avoidance of hyperextension in weight bearing and instead practicing a neutral elbow position.

Closing Remarks

In this chapter you learnt about two common postures of the elbow: flexed elbow and hyperextending elbow. The anatomical features of each are stated along with photographic examples and illustrations. The consequences of each posture are described, and for each pathology a table contains lists of shortened and lengthened muscles that will help you plan your treatments.

The following setup for display screen equipment will minimize postural stress in sitting.

Chair

- Sit with your hips and knees at approximately a 90-degree angle. This means sitting with thighs almost horizontal, level with your knees.
- The chair seat should be padded and at least 1 inch (2.5 cm) wider than your hips and thighs. It should slope down slightly.
- Sit back against the back of the chair unless the front edge of the seat presses into the backs of your knees. If the edge does press into the backs of your knees, change the chair for one with a seat of less depth. There should be two to three finger spaces between the edge of the chair and the backs of your knees.
- Adjust the height of your chair so that your feet are flat on the floor. If, once you have set up the rest of the equipment, it is necessary to raise your chair, use a footstool. Do not sit on your feet, twist your feet and ankles around the legs of the chair or sit cross-legged on the chair.
- If the chair has a lumbar support, make sure it is positioned correctly: against your lumbar spine rather than higher on your back or lower against your sacrum. Practice raising and lowering the level of the chair back to get comfortable.
- Adjust the tilt of the chair back so that you are not leaning too far back but at the same time are not sitting too erect. When using your chair, sit back into it rather than leaning forward towards your desk. If necessary, draw your chair closer to your desk.
- Remove the armrests of the chair if these prevent you from sitting close to your desk.
- The base of the chair should have five points that roll on casters.

Desk

- There should be adequate space beneath the desk and above your thighs.
- The desk itself and the area beneath the desk should be free from clutter, and any cables or wires should be fixed securely out of the way.
- Ensure that items used frequently are close at hand on your desk.

Keyboard and Mouse

- Centre the keyboard directly in front of you.
- Avoid positioning the keyboard too far from or too close to you. Either position, if prolonged, could stress your upper limb.
- Ensure the keyboard is free from glare.
- Work with your elbows close to your body and your arms and shoulders relaxed.

- Elbows should rest at approximately 90 to 100 degrees of flexion so that your forearms are almost horizontal.
- Wrists should be nearly straight, not overly flexed or extended, in line with your forearms.
- Choose a mouse that fits your hand comfortably and enables you to work with your wrist as straight as possible.
- Avoid holding your wrist in a deviated position when using the mouse.
- Avoid holding your arm in an outstretched position to use the mouse.
- Avoid resting your elbows or wrists on a hard surface.
- Hold the mouse lightly and tap keys on the keyboard lightly.

Monitor

- Position your monitor directly in front of you.
- Check that it is about an arm's length away.
- Position your monitor so that the top of the screen is approximately level with your eyes.
- Ensure the screen is free from glare.
- If necessary, use a document holder to prevent looking down and to one side whilst typing.

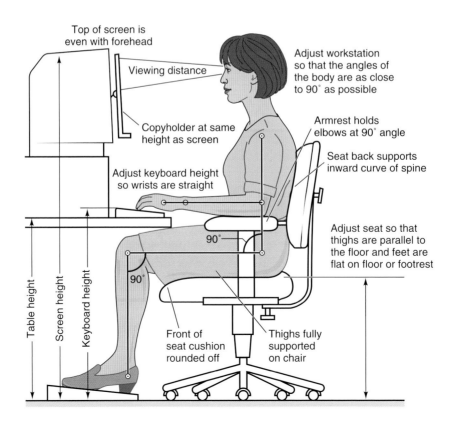

Chapter 1

Bloomfield, J., T.R. Ackland and B.C. Elliott. 1994. *Applied anatomy and biomechanics in sport*. Victoria, Australia: Blackwell Scientific.

Chin, M.K., K. Steininger, R.C.H. So, C.R. Clark and A.S.K. Wong. 1995. Physiological profiles and sport specific fitness of Asian elite squash players. *Br J Sports Med* 29 (3): 158-64.

Chansirinukor, W., D. Wilson, K. Grimmer and B. Danise. 2001. Effects of backpacks on students: measurement of cervical and shoulder posture. *Aust J of Physiother* 47 (2): 110-16.

Dehghani, L., M. Hashemi, R. Saboonchi, A. Hemalfar and A. Roonasi. 2012. Relationship between somatotype and some musculoskeletal deformities of girl students with Down syndrome. *Europ J Experimental Biol* 2 (4): 1209-13.

Forthomme, B., J-M Crielaard and J-L Croisier. 2008. Scapular positioning in athlete's shoulder. *Sports Med* 38 (5): 369-86.

Grabara, M. 2012. Analysis of body postures between young football players and their untrained peers. *Hum Mov* 13 (2): 120-26.

Hennessy, L., and A.W.S. Watson. 1993. Flexibility and posture assessment in relation to hamstring injury. *Br J Med*. 27 (4): 243-46.

Herbert, R.D., and R.J. Balnave. 1993. The effect of position of immobilisation on resting length, resting stiffness, and weight of the soleus muscle of the rabbit. *J Orthop Res* 11 (3): 358–66.

Heslinga, J.W., G. te Kronnie and P.A. Huijing. 1995. Growth and immobilization effects on sarcomeres: A comparison between gastrocnemius and soleus muscles of the adult rat. *Eur J Appl Physiol Occup Physiol* 70 (1): 49–57.

Oyama, S., J.B. Myers, C.A. Wessinger, R.D. Ricci and S.M Lephart. 2008. Asymmetric resting scapular posture in healthy overhead athletes *J of Athletic Training* 43 (6): 565-70.

Pourbehzadi, M., H. Sadeghi, H.A. Alinehad and L.S. Rad. 2012. The relationship between posture and somatotype and certain biomechanical parameters of Iran women's national dragon boat team. *Annals of Biological Research* 3 (7): 3657-62.

Spector, S.A. C.P. Simard, M. Fournier, E. Sternlicht and V.R. Edgerton. 1982. Architectural alterations of rat hind-limb skeletal muscles immobilized at different lengths. *Exp Neurol* 76 (1): 94–110.

Tinkle, B.T. 2008. *Joint hypermobility*. Niles, IL: Left Paw Press.

Travell, J., and D.L. Simons. 1999. *Myofascial pain and dysfunction: The trigger point manual*. Vol. 1, 2nd ed. Philadelphia: Lippincott Williams & Williams.

Watson, A.W.A. 1997. Posture: Introduction and its relationship to participation in sports *Rev. Fisioter. Uni. São Paulo* 4 (1): 1-46.

Chapter 2

American Academy of Orthopaedic Surgeons. 2007. How to sit at a computer. http://orthoinfo.aaos.org/topic.cfm?topic=A00261. Accessed December 21, 2014.

American Chiropractic Association. 2014. Tips to maintain good posture. www.acatoday.org/content_css.cfm?CID=1452. Accessed December 21, 2014.

American College of Sports Medicine. 2011. Quantity and quality of exercise for developing and maintaining cardiorespiratory, musculoskeletal, and neuromuscular fitness in apparently healthy adults: Guidance for prescribing exercise. *Medicine and Science in Sports & Exercise.* DOI:10.1249/MSS.0b013e318213fefb.

Bloomfield, J., T.R. Ackland and B.C. Elliott. 1994. *Applied anatomy and biomechanics in sport.* Victoria, Australia: Blackwell Scientific.

Chaitow, L. 2001. *Muscle energy techniques.* London: Churchill Livingstone.

Chartered Society of Physiotherapists. 2013. Perfect posture. file:///Users/ul8/Downloads/csp_sitatdesk_postcards_2013.pdf. Accessed December 21, 2014.

Chartered Society of Physiotherapy and Fitness Industry Association Joint Working Party. 2011. Guidance on the referral of patients between physiotherapists and fitness instructors Produced by the Chartered Society of Physiotherapy and Fitness Industry Association Joint Working Party. 2011. file:///Users/ul8/Downloads/csp_guidance_referral_patients_physios_fitness_instructors_2011_0.pdf. Accessed January 26, 2015.

College of Occupational Therapists and Association of Chartered Physiotherapists in Neurology. 2015. Splinting for the prevention and correction of contractures in adults with neurological dysfunction. London: College of Occupational Therapists. www.acpin.net/Splinting_Guidelines/Splinting_Guidelines.pdf.

Donatelli, R. 1987. Abnormal biomechanics of the foot and ankle. *J Orthop Sports Phys Ther* 9 (1): 11-16.

Duncan, R. 2014. *Myofascial release.* Champaign, IL: Human Kinetics.

Earls, J. and T. Myers. 2010. *Fascial release for structural balance.* England: Lotus.

Fawdington, R.A., B. Johnson and N.T. Kiely. 2013. Lower limb deformity assessment and correction. *Orthopaedics and Trauma* 28 (1): 33-40.

Gross, M.T. 1995. Lower quarter screening for skeletal malalignment—suggestions for orthotics and shoewear. *J Orthop Sports Phys Ther* 21 (6): 389-405.

Guimond, S., and W. Massrieh. 2012. Intricate correlation between body posture, personality train and incidence of body pain: A cross-referential study report. *PLoS ONE* 7, no. 5. Accessed December 15, 2014. DOI:10.1371/journal.pone.0037450.

Hanten, W.P., S.L. Olson, N.L. Butts and A.L. Nowicki. 2000. Effectiveness of a home programme of ischemic pressure followed by sustained stretch for treatment of myofascial trigger points. *Phys Ther* 80 (10): 997-1003.

Health & Safety Executive. 2013. Working with display screen equipment (DSE). www.hse.gov.uk/pubns/indg36.pdf. Accessed December 21, 2014.

Hertling, D., and R.M. Kessler. 2006. *Management of common musculoskeletal disorders.* 4th ed. Philadelphia: Lippincott Williams & Wilkins.

Heslinga, J.W., G. te Kronnie and P.A. Huijing. 1995. Growth and immobilization effects on sarcomeres: A comparison between gastrocnemius and soleus muscles of the adult rat. *Eur J Appl Physiol Occup Physiol* 70 (1): 49–57.

Holey, E., and E. Cook. 2003. Evidence-based therapeutic massage: A practical guide for therapists. 2nd ed. Edinburgh. Churchill Livingstone.

Huguenin, L.K. 2004. Myofascial trigger points: the current evidence. *Physical Therapy in Sport* 5 (1): 2-12.

Jacobs, C.A., and A.D. Sciascia. 2011. Factors that influence the efficacy of stretching programmes for patients with hypomobility. *Sports Health* 3 (6): 520-23.

Jarvis, H.L., C.J. Nester, R.K. Jones, A. Williams and P.D. Bowden. 2012. Inter-assessor reliability of practice based biomechanical assessment of the foot and ankle. *Journal of Foot and Ankle Research* 5:14. DOI: 10.1186/1757-1146-5-14. Accessed December 22, 2014.

Johnson, J. 2009. *Soft tissue release*. Champaign, IL: Human Kinetics.

Johnson, J. 2010. *Deep tissue massage*. Champaign, IL: Human Kinetics.

Johnson, J. 2012. *Postural assessment*. Champaign, IL: Human Kinetics.

Johnson, J. 2014. *Therapeutic stretching*. Champaign, IL: Human Kinetics.

Kendall, F.P., E.K. McCreary. 1983. *Muscles: Testing and function*. 3rd ed. Baltimore: Lippincott Williams and Wilkins.

Kendall, F.P., E.K. McCreary and P.G. Provance. 1993. *Muscles: Testing and function*. 4th ed. Baltimore: Lippincott Williams and Wilkins.

Kidd, M.O., C.H. Bond and M.L. Bell. 2011. Patients' perspectives of patient-centredness as important in musculoskeletal physiotherapy interactions: A qualitative study *Physiotherapy* 97 (2): 154-162.

Langendoen, J., and K. Sertel. 2011. *Kinesiology taping*. Ontario, Canada: Rose.

Lavelle, E.D., W. Lavelle and H.S. Smith. 2007. Myofascial trigger points. *Anesthesiol Clin* 25 (4): 841-51.

Lee, L.J. 2013. Thoracic ring control: A missing link? MPA *In Touch* 4: 13F16.

Milroy, P., and G. O'Neil. 2000. Factors affecting compliance to chiropractic prescribed home exercise: a review of the literature. *J Can Chiropr Assoc* 44 (3): 141-48.

National Institutes of Health. 2014. Ergonomics program: The computer workstation. www.ors.od.nih.gov/sr/dohs/Documents/ORS_Ergonomics_Poster_Rd5.pdf. Accessed December 21, 2014.

Panel on Musculoskeletal Disorders and the Workplace Commission on Behavioral and Social Sciences and Education National Research Council and Institute of Medicine. 2001. Musculoskeletal disorders and the workplace: Low back and upper extremities. www.nap.edu/openbook.php?isbn=0309072840. Accessed December 15, 2014.

Randall, K.E., and I.R. McEwen. 2000. Writing patient centred goals. *Physical Therapy* 80 (12): 1197-1203.

Sackett, D.L. 1996. Evidenced based medicine: What it is and what it isn't. *BMJ* 312 (7023): 71-2.

Sanders, B., A.A. Blackburn and B. Boucher. 2013. Preparticipation screening: The sports physical therapy perspective. *Int J of Sports Physic Ther* 8 (2): 180-93.

Sarasohn-Kahn, J. (Ed.) 2013. *Personal health information technology—paradigm for providers and patients to transform healthcare through patient engagement*. Healthcare Information and Management Systems. www.himss.org/ResourceLibrary/GenResourceReg.aspx?ItemNumber=22235. Accessed November 2014.

Simons, D.G. 2002. Understanding effective treatments of myofascial trigger points. *Journal of Bodywork and Movement Therapies* 6 (2): 81-88.

Sluijs, E.M., G.J. Kok and J. van der Zee. 1993. Correlates of exercise compliance in physical therapy. *Phys Ther* 73 (11): 771-82.

Society of Sports Therapists. 2013. What is sports therapy? www.society-of-sports-therapists.org/index.php/public_information/what-is-sports-therapy. Accessed January 28, 2015.

Tidy, N.M. 1944. *Massage & remedial exercises in medical and surgical conditions*. 6th ed. Bristol, UK: Wright.

Troyanovich, S.J., D.E. Harrison and D.D. Harrison. 1998. The structural rehabilitation of the spine and posture: Rational for treatment beyond the resolution of symptoms. *J of Manipulative & Physiol Ther* 21 (1): 37-50.

Verhoef, M.J., L.C. Vanderheyden, T. Dryden, D. Mallory and M.A. Ware. 2006. Evaluating complementary and alternative medicine interventions: In search of appropriate patient-centered outcome measures. *BMC Complementary and Alternative Medicine* 6: 38. DOI: 10.1186/1472-6882-6-38.

Woodard, C.J., and M. J. Berry. 2001. Enhancing adherence to prescribed exercise: Structured behavioural interventions in clinical exercise programs. *J Cardiopulm Rehabil* 21 (4): 201-9.

Chapter 3

Caneiro, J.P., P. O'Sullivan, A. Burnett, A. Barach, D. O'Neil, O. Tveit, and K. Olafsdottir. 2010. The influence of different sitting postures on head/neck posture and muscle activity. *Man Ther* 15 (1): 54-60.

Chansirinukor, W., D. Wilson, K. Grimmer and B. Danise. 2001. Effects of backpacks on students: Measurement of cervical and shoulder posture. *Aust J of Physiother* 47 (2): 110-16.

Falla, D. 2004. Unravelling the complexity of muscle impairment in chronic neck pain. *Man Ther* 9 (3): 125-33.

Falla, D., G.A. Jull and P.W. Hodges. 2004. Patients with neck pain demonstrate reduced electromyographic activity of the deep cervical neck flexor muscles during performance of the craniocervical flexion test. *Spine* 29 (19): 2108-14.

Grimmer, K., and P. Trott. 1998. The association between cervical excursion angles and cervical short flexor muscle endurance. *Aust J Physiother* 44 (3): 201-7.

Gupta, B.D., S. Aggarwal, B. Gupta, M. Gupta and N. Gupta. 2013. Effect of deep cervical flexor training vs. conventional isometric training on forward head posture, pain, neck disability index in dentists suffering from chronic neck pain. *J Clin Diag Res* 7 (10): 2261-64.

Jull, G.A., S.P. O'Leary and D.L. Falla. 2008. Clinical assessment of the deep cervical flexor muscles: The craniocervical flexion test. *J Manipulative Physiol Ther* 31 (7): 525-33.

National Institute of Neurological Disorders and Stroke. 2014. *Dystonias factsheet*. www.ninds. nih.gov/disorders/dystonias/detail_dystonias.htm. Accessed July 30, 2014.

Noh, H.J., J.H. Shim and Y.J. Jeon. 2013. Effects of neck stabilization exercises on neck and shoulder muscle activation in adults with forward head posture. *JDCTA* 7 (12): 492-98.

Raine, S., and L. Twomey. 1994. Posture of the head, shoulders and thoracic spine in comfortable erect standing. *Aust J Physiother* 40 (1): 25-32.

Waldman, S.D. 2008. *Atlas of uncommon pain syndromes*. 2nd ed. Philadelphia: Saunders.

Wang, R., E.R. Snoey, R.C. Clements, H.G. Hern and D. Price. 2006. Effect of head rotation on vascular anatomy of the neck: An ultrasound study. *J Emerg Med* 31 (3): 283-6.

Yoo, W.G. 2013. Effect of neck retraction taping (NRT) on forward head posture and the upper trapezius muscle during computer work. *J Phys Ther Sci* 25 (5): 581-82.

Chapter 4

Caneiro, J.P., P. O'Sullivan, A. Burnett, A. Barach, D. O'Neil, O. Tveit, and K. Olafsdottir. 2010. The influence of different sitting postures on head/neck posture and muscle activity. *Man Ther* 15 (1): 54-60.

Crawford, H.J., and G.A. Jull. 1993. The influence of thoracic posture and movement on range of arm elevation. *Physiotherapy Theory and Practice* 9 (3): 143-48. Accessed July 2014. DOI: 10.3109/09593989309047453.

Gertzbein, S.D., D. Macmichael and M. Tile. 1982. Harrington instrumentation as a method of fixation in fractures of the spine *J Bone Joint Surg Br* 64 (5): 526-29.

Grabara, M., and J. Szopa. 2011. Effects of hatha yoga on the shaping of the antero-posterior curvature of the spine. *Human Movement* 12 (3): 259-63.

Greendale, G.A., M.H. Huang, A.S. Karlamangla, L. Seeger and S. Crawford. 2009. Yoga decreases kyphosis in senior women and men with adult-onset hyperkyphosis: Results of a randomized controlled trial. *J Am Geriatr Soc* 57 (9): 1569-79.

Gulbahar, S., E. Sahin, M. Baydar, C. Bircan, R. Kizil, M. Manisali, E. Akalin and O. Peker. 2006. Hypermobility syndrome increases the risk for low bone mass. *Clin Rheumatol* 25 (4): 511-14.

Harrison, D.E., C.J. Colloca, D.D. Harrison, T.J. Janik, J.W. Haas and T.S. Keller. 2005. Anterior thoracic posture increases thoracolumbar disc loading. *Eur Spine J* 14: 234-42.

Lee, L.J., M.W. Coppleters and P.W. Hodges. 2005. Differential activation of the thoracic multifidus and longissimus thoracis during trunk rotation. *Spine* 30 (8): 870-76.

Lee, L.J. 2008. Is it time for a closer look at the thorax? *In Touch* 1: 13-16.

Lewis, J.S., C. Wright and A. Green. 2005. Subacromial impingement syndrome: The effect of changing posture on shoulder range of movement. *J Orthop Sports Phys Ther* 35 (2): 72-87.

O'Gorman, H., and G. Jull. 1987. Thoracic kyphosis and mobility: The effect of age. *Physiotherapy Theory and Practice* 3 (4): 152-62.

Raine, S., and L. Twomey. 1994. Posture of the head, shoulders and thoracic spine in comfortable erect standing. *Aust J Physiother* 40 (1): 25-32.

Chapter 5

Adams, M.A., and W.C. Hutton. 1980. The effect of posture on the role of apophyseal joints in resisting intervertebral compressive forces. *J Bone Joint Surg Br* 62 (3): 358-62.

Adams, M.A., and W.C. Hutton. 1985. The effect of posture on the lumbar spine. *J Bone Joint Surg Br* 67 (4): 625-29.

Been, E., and L. Kalichman. 2014. Lumbar lordosis. *The Spine Journal* 14 (1): 87-97. DOI: http://dx.doi.org/10.1016/j.spinee.2013.07.464. Accessed May 2014.

Bloomfield, J., T.R. Ackland and B.C. Elliott. 1994. *Applied anatomy and biomechanics in sport*. Victoria, Australia: Blackwell Scientific.

Caneiro, J.P., P. O'Sullivan, A. Burnett, A. Barach, D. O'Neil, O. Tveit, and K. Olafsdottir. 2010. The influence of different sitting postures on head/neck posture and muscle activity. *Man Ther* 15 (1): 54-60.

Capson, A.C., J. Nashed and L. McLean. 2011. The effect of lumbopelvic posture on pelvic floor muscle activation and intravaginal pressure generation in continent women. *J Electromyogr Kinesiol* (1): 166-77.

Duncan, R. 2014. *Myofascial release*. Champaign, IL: Human Kinetics.

Earls, J., and T. Myers. 2010. *Fascial release for structural balance*. Chichester, UK: Lotus.

Fernard, R., and D.E. Fox. 1985. Evaluation of lumbar lordosis: A prospective and retrospective study. *Spine* 10 (9): 799-803.

Gajdosik, R. 1997. Hamstring stretching and posture. Letter to the editor. *Phys Ther* 77: 438-39.

Halski, T., L. Slupska, R. Dymarek, J. Bartnicki, U. Halska, A. Król, K. Paprocka-Borowicz, J. Dembowski, R. Zdrojowry and K. Ptaszkowski. 2014. Evaluation of bioelectrical activity of pelvic floor muscles and synergistic muscles depending on orientation of pelvis in menopausal women with symptoms of stress urinary incontinence: A preliminary observational study. *Biomed Research International*. Article ID 274938. DOI: 10.1155/2014/274938. Accessed June 2014.

Harrison, D.E., R. Cailliet, D.D. Harrison, T.J. Janik and B. Holland. 2002. Changes in sagittal lumbar configuration with a new method of extension traction: Nonrandomized clinical control trial. *Arch Phys Med Rehabil* 83 (11): 1585-91.

Harrison, D.E., C.J. Colloca, D.D. Harrison, T.J. Janik, J.W. Haas and T.S. Keller. 2005. Anterior thoracic posture increases thoracolumbar disc loading. *Eur Spine J* 14: 234-42.

Hashimoto, K., K. Miyamoto, T. Yanagawa, R. Hattori, T. Aoki, T. Matsuoka, T. Ohno and K. Shimizu. 2013. Lumbar corsets can decrease lumbar motion in golf swing. *Journal of Sports Science and Medicine* 12 (1): 80-87.

Kendall, F.P., E.K. McCreary and P.G. Provance. 1993. *Muscles: Testing and function*. 4th ed. Baltimore: Lippincott Williams and Wilkins.

Kim, M.H., and W.G. Yoo. 2014. Effects of inclined treadmill walking on pelvic anterior tilt angle, hamstring muscle length, and trunk muscle endurance of seated workers with flat-back syndrome. *J Phys Ther Sci* 26 (6): 855-56.

Li, Y., P.W. McClure, and N. Pratt. 1996. The effect of hamstring muscle stretching on standing posture and on lumbar and hip motions during forward bending. *Phys Ther* 76 (8): 836-45.

Majeske, C., and C. Buchanan. 1984. Quantitative description of two sitting postures: With and without lumbar support pillow. *Phys Ther* 64 (10): 1531-35.

Russell, B.S., K.T Muhlenkamp, C.M. Hoiriis and C.M. DeSimone. 2012. Measurement of lumbar lordosis in static standing posture with and without high-heeled shoes. *J Chiropr Med* 11 (3): 145–53.

Scannell, J.P., and S.M. McGill. 2003. Lumbar posture—should it, and can it, be modified? A study of passive tissue stiffness and lumbar position during activities of daily living. *Phys Ther* 83 (10): 907-17.

Silva, A.M., G.R. de Siqueira and G.A. da Silva. 2013. Implications of high-heeled shoes on body posture of adolescents. *Rev Paul Pediatr* 32 (2): 265-71.

Smith, R.L., and D.B. Mell. 1987. The effects of prone extension exercise on lumbar extension range of motion. *Phys Ther* 67 (10): 1517-21.

Sparrey, C.J., J.F. Bailey, M. Safaee, A.J. Clark, V. Lafage, F. Schwab, J.S. Smith and C.P. Ames. 2014. Etiology of lumbar lordosis and its pathophysiology: A review of the evolution of lumbar lordosis, and the mechanics and biology of lumbar degeneration. *Journal of Neurosurgery* 36 (5): 1-16. DOI: 10.3171/2014.1.focus13551. Accessed July 2014.

Tüzün, Ç., I. Yorulmaz, A. Cindaş and S. Vatan. 1999. Low back pain and posture. *Clin Rheumatol* 18 (4): 308-12.

Yoo, W.G. 2013. Effect of individual strengthening exercises for anterior pelvic tilt muscles on back pain, pelvic angle, and lumbar ROMs of a LBP patient with flat back. *J Phys Ther Sci* 25 (10): 1357-58.

Chapter 6

British Scoliosis Society. 2008. Patient information. www.britscoliosissoc.org.uk/article. asp?article=2. Accessed September 3, 2014.

Curtin M., and M.M. Lowery. 2014. Musculoskeletal modelling of muscle activation and applied external forces for the correction of scoliosis.. *Journal of NeuroEngineering and Rehabilitation* 11(52). DOI: 10.1186/1743-0003-11-52.

Gielen, J.L., and E. Van den Eede. 2008. FIMS Position statement: Scoliosis and sports participation. *International SportMed Journal* 9 (3): 131-40.

Gogala, A. 2014. Correction of scoliosis in adulthood without surgery. www2.pms-lj.si/bibliag/scoliosis.pdf. Accessed August 31, 2014. Original article published in Slovenian in two parts: Gogala, A. 2014. Zdravljenje skolioze v odrasli dobi brez operacije. 1. del: Zgodba *Proteus*. 76(8): 358-365 and Gogala, A. 2014. Zdravljenje skolioze v odrasli dobi brez operacije. 2. del: Razprava *Proteus*. 76(9): 405-412.

Hawes, M.C., and J.P. O'Brien. 2006. The transformation of spinal curvature into spinal deformity: pathological processes and implications for treatment. www.scoliosisjournal.com/content/1/1/3. Accessed September 2014.

National Scoliosis Foundation. 2014. Information and support. www.scoliosis.org/info.php. Accessed September 2014.

Negrini, A., H. Verzini, S. Parzini, A. Negrini, A. and S. Negrini. 2001. Role of physical exercise in the treatment of mild idiopathic adolescent scoliosis: Review of the literature. *Eur Med Phys* 37: 181-90.

Pourbehzadi, M., H. Sadeghi, H.A. Alinehad and L.S. Rad. 2012. The relationship between posture and somatotype and certain biomechanical parameters of Iran women's national dragon boat team. *Annals of Biological Research* 3 (7): 3657-62.

Scoliosis Association (UK). 2014. Complementary therapies. www.sauk.org.uk/about-scoliosis/complementary-therapies.html. Accessed September 2014.

Scoliosis Research Society. 2015. Patient and family. www.srs.org/patient_and_family. Accessed September 2014.

Solberg, G. 2008. *Postural disorders and musculoskeletal dysfunction: Diagnosis, prevention and treatment*. 2nd ed. Edinburgh/New York: Churchill Livingstone.

Vialle, R., C. Thévenin-Lemoine and P. Mary. 2013. Neuromuscular scoliosis. *Orthop Traumatol Surg Res* 99 (1): S124-S39.

Watson, A.W.A. 1997. Posture: Introduction and its relationship to participation in sports. *Rev. Fisioter. Uni. São Paulo* 4 (1): 1-46.

Weinstein, S.L., D.C. Zavala and I.V. Ponsetti. 1981. Idiopathic scoliosis: Long-term follow-up and prognosis in untreated patients. *J Bone Joint Surg Am* 63 (5): 702-12.

Weinstein, S.L., L.A. Dolan, K.F. Spratt, K.K. Peterson, M.J. Spoonmore and I.V. Ponseti. 2003. Health and function of patients with untreated idiopathic scoliosis: A 50-year natural history study. *JAMA* 289 (5): 559-67.

Yadla, S., M.G. Maltenfort, J.K. Ratliff and J.S. Harrop. 2010. Adult scoliosis surgery outcomes: A systematic review. *Neurosurgical Focus* 28 (3): E3: 1-7.

Chapter 7

Adams, M.A., and W.C. Hutton. 1985. The effect of posture on the lumbar spine. *J Bone Joint Surg Br* 67 (4): 625-29.

Bloomfield, J., T.R. Ackland and B.C. Elliott. 1994. *Applied anatomy and biomechanics in sport*. Victoria, Australia: Blackwell Scientific.

Bohannon, R., R. Gajdosik and B.F. LeVeau. 1985. Contribution of pelvic and lower limb motion to increases in the angle of passive straight leg raising. *Phy Ther* 65 (4): 474-76.

Boulay, C., C. Tardieu, C. Bénaim, J. Hecquet, C. Marty, D. Prat-Pradal, J. Legaye, G. Duval-Beaupère and J. Pélissier. 2006. Three-dimensional study of pelvic asymmetry on anatomical specimens and its clinical perspective. *J Anat* 208 (1): 21-33.

Brunstromm, S. 2012. *Clinical kinesiology*. 2012. 6th ed. Philadelphia: Davis.

Cohen, S.P. 2005. Sacroiliac joint pain: A comprehensive review of anatomy, diagnosis, and treatment. *Anesthesia & Analgesia*. 101 (5): 1440-1453.

Cooperstein, R. and M. Lew. 2009. The relationship between pelvic torsion and anatomical leg length discrepancy: A review of the literature. *J Chiropr Med* 8 (3): 107-13.

Day, J.W., G.L. Smidt and T. Lehmann. 1984. Effect of pelvic tilt on standing posture. *Phys Ther* 64 (4): 510-16.

Deckert, J.L. 2009. Improving pelvic alignment. *IADMS Bulletin for Teachers* 1 (1): 11-12.

Gnat, R., E. Saulicz, M. Bialy and P. Klaptocz. 2009. Does pelvic asymmetry always mean pathology? Analysis of mechanical factors leading to the asymmetry. *J Hum Kinet* 21: 23-35.

Kapandji, A.I., 2008. *The physiology of the joints: Volume 3 the spinal column, pelvic girdle and head*. London: Churchill Livingstone.

Kendall, F.P., E.K. McCreary and P.G. Provance. 1993. *Muscles: Testing and function.* 4th ed. Baltimore: Lippincott Williams and Wilkins.

Klingensmith, R.D., and C.L. Blum. 2003. The relationship between pelvic block placement and radiographic pelvic analysis. *Journal of Chiropractic Medicine* 2 (3): 102-106.

Levangie, P.K., and C.C. Norkin. 2001. *Joint structure and function: A comprehensive analysis.* Philadelphia: Davis.

Lee, J.H., W.G. Woo, M.H. Kim, J.S. Oh, K.S. Lee and J.T. Han. 2014. Effect of posterior pelvic tilt taping on women with sacroiliac joint pain during active straight leg raising who habitually wore high-heeled shoes: A preliminary study. *Journal of Manipulative and Physiological Therapeutics* 37 (4): 260-68.

Lippold C., G. Danesh, G. Hoppe, B. Drerup, and L. Hackenberg. 2007. Trunk inclination, pelvic tilt and pelvic rotation in relation to the craniofacial morphology in adults. *The Angle Orthodontist,* 77 (1): 29-35.

López-Miñarro, P.A., J.M. Muyor, F. Belmonte and F. Alacid. 2012. Acute effects of hamstring stretching on sagittal spinal curvatures and pelvic tilt. *J Hum Kinet* 31: 69-78.

Scannell, J.P., and S.M. McGill. 2003. Lumbar posture—should it, and can it, be modified? A study of passive tissue stiffness and lumbar position during activities of daily living. *Phys Ther* 83 (10): 907-17.

Viggiani, D., M. Nagouchi, K. M. Gruveski, D. De Carvalho and J. P. Callaghan. (2014). The effect of wallet thickness on spine sitting posture, seat interface pressure, and perceived discomfort during sitting. *IIE Transactions on Occupational Ergonomics and Human Factors.* DOI: 10.1080/21577323.2014.962712.

Chapter 8

Alter, M.J. 2004. *The science of flexibility.* Champaign, IL: Human Kinetics.

American Academy of Orthopaedic Surgeons. 2014. Adult acquired flatfoot. http://orthoinfo. aaos.org/topic.cfm?topic=A00173. Accessed November 3, 2014.

American College of Foot and Ankle Surgeons. 2014a. Cavus foot (high-arched foot). www. foothealthfacts.org/footankleinfo/cavus-foot.htm?terms=high%20arched%20foot. Accessed November 2014.

American College of Foot and Ankle Surgeons. 2014b. Flexible flatfoot. www.foothealthfacts. org/footankleinfo/flatfoot.htm. Accessed November 2014.

American College of Foot and Ankle Surgeons. 2014c. Common disorders of the Achilles tendon. www.foothealthfacts.org/footankleinfo/achilles-tendon.htm. Accessed November 2014.

Banwell, H.A., S. Mackintosh and D. Thewlis. 2014. Foot orthoses for adults with flexible pes planus: A systematic review. *Journal of Foot and Ankle Research.* 7 (23). www.jfootankleres. com. DOI: 10.1186/1757-1146-7-23. Accessed November 2014,

Betsch, M., J. Schneppendahl, L. Dor, P. Jungbluth, J.P. Grassmann, J. Windolf, S. Thelen, M. Hakimi, W. Rapp and M. Wild. 2011. Influence of foot positions on the spine and pelvis. *Arthritis Care Res* 63 (12): 1758-65.

Beynnon, B.D., D.F. Murphy and D.M. Alosa. 2002. Predictive factors for lateral ankle sprains: a literature review. *J Athl Train* 37 (4): 376-380.

Bloomfield, J., T.R. Ackland and B.C. Elliott. 1994. *Applied anatomy and biomechanics in sport.* Victoria, Australia: Blackwell Scientific.

Burns, J., K.B. Landorf, M.M. Ryan, J. Crosbie and R.A. Ouvrier. 2007. Interventions for the prevention and treatment of pes cavus. Cochrane Database of Systematic Reviews 17 (4) CD006154. DOI: 10.1002/14651858.CD006154.pub2.

Cerejo, R., D.D. Dunlop, S. Cahue, D. Channin, J. Song and L. Sharma. 2002. The influence of alignment on risk of knee osteoarthritis progression according to baseline stage of disease. *Arthritis Rheum* 46 (10): 2632-36.

Clementz, B.G. 1988. Tibial torsion measured in normal adults. *Acta Orthop Scand* 59 (4): 441-42.

Cooperstein, R., and M. Lew, 2009. The relationship between pelvic torsion and anatomical leg length discrepancy: a review of the literature. *J Chiropr Med* 8 (3): 107-13.

Corps, N., A.H. Robinson, R.L. Harrall, N.C. Avery, C.A. Curry, B.L. Hazleman and G.P. Riley. 2012. Changes in matrix protein biochemistry and the expression of mRNA encoding matrix proteins and metalloproteinases in posterior tibialis tendinopathy. *Ann Rheum Dis* 71 (5): 746-52.

Devan, M.R., L.S. Pescatello, P. Faghri and J. Anderson. 2004. A prospective study of overuse knee injuries among female athletes with muscle imbalances and structural abnormalities. *Journal of Athletic Training* 39 (3): 263-67.

Donatelli, R. 1987. Abnormal biomechanics of the foot and ankle. *J Orthop Sports Phys Ther* 9 (1): 11-16.

Fan, Y., Y. Fan, Z. Li, C. Lv and D. Luo. 2011. Natural gaits of the non-pathological flat foot and high-arched foot. *PLoS ONE* 6 (3): e17749. DOI:10.1371/journal.pone.0017749. Accessed November 2014.

Fish, D.J., and C.S. Kosta. 1998. Genu recurvatum: Identification of three distinct mechanical profiles. *J of Prosthetics and Orthotics* 10 (2): 26-32.

Fowler, R.P. 2004. Recommendations for management of uncomplicated back pain in workers' compensation system: A focus on functional restoration. *J Chiropr Med* 3 (4): 129-37.

Gandhi, S., R.K. Singla, J.S. Kullar, G. Agnihotri, V. Mehta, R.K. Suri and G. Rath. 2014. Human tibial torsion—morphometric assessment and clinical relevance. *Biomed J* 37 (1): 10-13.

Gross, M.T. 1995. Lower quarter screening for skeletal malalignment—suggestions for orthotics and shoewear. *J Orthop Sports Phys Ther* 21 (6): 389-405.

Hagedorn, T.J., A.B. Dufour, J.L. Riskowski, H.J. Hillstrom, H.B. Menz, V.A. Casey and M.T. Hannan. 2013. Foot disorder, foot posture, and foot function: The Framington foot study. *PLoS One* 8 (9) e74364. DOI: 10.1371/journal.pone.0074364. Accessed September 2014.

Hartman, A.K., Murer, R.A. de Bie and E.D. de Bruin. 2009. The effect of a foot gymnastic exercise programme on gait performance in older adults: A randomised controlled trial. *Disabil Rehabil* 31 (25): 2101-10. DOI: 10.3109/09638280902927010. Accessed July 2014

Hicks, J., A. Arnold, F. Anderson, M. Schwartz and S. Delp. 2007. The effect of excessive tibial torsion on the capacity of muscles to extend the hip and knee during single-limb stance. *Gait Posture* 26 (4): 546-52.

Hughes, J., P. Clark and L. Klenerman. 1990. The importance of toes in walking. *J Bone Joint Surg Br* 72 (2): 245-51.

Inman, V.T. 1966. Human locomotion. *Cana. Med Ass J* 94 (4): 1047-54.

Kendall, F.P., E.K. McCreary and P.G. Provance. 1993. *Muscles: Testing and function.* 4th ed. Baltimore: Lippincott Williams and Wilkins.

Kerrigan, D.C., L.C. Deming and M.K. Holden. 1996. Knee recurvatum in gait: A study of associated knee biomechanics. *Arch Phys Med Rehabil* 77 (7): 645-50.

Knight, I. 2011. *A guide to living with hypermobility syndrome.* 2011. Philadelphia: Singing Dragon.

Kohls-Gatzoulis, J., J.C. Angel, D. Singh, F. Haddad, J. Livingstone and G. Berry. 2004. Tibialis posterior dysfunction: A common and treatable cause of adult acquired flatfoot. *BMJ* 329 (7478): 1328-33.

Kouyoumdjian, P., R. Coulomb, T. Sanchez and G. Asencio. 2012. Clinical evaluation of hip joint rotation range of motion in adults. *Orthop Traumatol Surg Res* 98 (1): 17-23.

Langendoen, J., and K. Sertel. 2011. *Kinesiology taping*. Ontario, Canada: Robert Rose.

Levangie, P.K., and C.C. Norkin. 2001. *Joint structure and function: A comprehensive analysis*. Philadelphia: Davis.

Levinger, P., H.B. Menz, M.R. Fotoohabadi, J.A. Feller, J.R. Bartlett and N.R. Bergman. 2010. Foot posture in people with medial compartment knee osteoarthritis. *Journal of Foot and Ankle Research* 3 (29). DOI: 10.1186/1757-1146-3-29. Accessed September 2014.

Levinger, P., H.B. Menz, A.D. Morrow, J.A. Feller, H.R. Bartlett and N.R. Bergman. 2012. Foot kinematics in people with medial compartment knee osteoarthritis. *Rheumatology (Oxford)* 51 (12): 2191-98.

Loudon, J.K., H.L. Goist and K.L. Loudon. 1998. Genu recurvatum syndrome. *J Orthop Sports Phys Ther* 27 (5): 361-367.

Lun, V., W.H. Meeuwisse, P. Stergiou and D. Stefanyshyn. 2004. Relation between running injury and static lower limb alignment in recreational runners. *Br J Sports Med* 38: 576-80.

Luque-Suarez, A., G. Gijon-Nogueron, F.J. Baron-Lopez, M.T. Labajos-Manzanares, J. Hush and M.J. Hancock. 2014. Effects of kinesiotaping on foot posture in participants with pronated foot: A quasi-randomised, double-blind study. *Physiotherapy* 100 (1): 36-40.

Magee, D. J. 2002. *Orthopedic physical assessment.* 4th ed. Philadelphia: Saunders.

McWilliams, D.F., S. Doherty, R.A. Maciewicz, K.R. Muir, W. Zhang and M. Doherty. 2010. Self-reported knee and foot alignments in early adult life and risk of osteoarthritis. *Arthritis Care Res* 62 (4): 489-95.

Malvankar, S., Khan, W., Mahapatra, A and G.S.E. Dowd. 2012. How effective are lateral wedge orthotics in treating medial compartment osteoarthritis of the knee? A systematic review of the recent literature. *Open Orthotics Journal* 6 (Suppl 3: M8): 2012: 544-547. DOI: 10.2174/1874325001206010544. Accessed September 2014.

Manoli, A. and B. Graham. 2005. The subtle cavus foot, the "underpronator: A review: *Foot Ankle Int* 26 (3): 256-263.

Mullaji, A.B., A.K. Sharma, S.V. Marawar and A.F. Kohli. 2008. Tibial torsion in non-arthritic Indian adults: a computer tomography study of 100 limbs. *Indian J Orthop* 42 (3): 309-13.

Myerson, M.S. 1996. Adult acquired flatfoot deformity: Treatment of dysfunction of the posterior tibial tendon. *Instr Course* 46: 393-505.

Neumann, D.A. 2010. Kinesiology of the hip: A focus on muscular actions. *J Orthop Sports Phys Ther* 40 (2): 82-94.

Perkins, G. 1947. Pes planus or instability of the longitudinal arch. *Proc Royal Soc Med* 41 (1): 31-40.

Riegger-Krugh, C., and J.J. Keysor. 1996. Skeletal malalignments of the lower quarter: Correlated and compensatory motions and postures. *J Orthop Sports Physical Therapy* 23 (2): 164-70.

Ritchie, G.W., and H.A. Keim. 1964. A radiographic analysis of major foot deformities. *Can Med Assoc J* 91 (16): 840-44.

Rodrigues, P.T., A.F. Ferreira, R.M. Pereira, E. Bonfá, E.F. Borba and R. Fuller. 2008. Effectiveness of medial-wedge insole treatment for valgus knee osteoarthritis. *Arthritis Rheum* 15 (59): 603-08.

Samaei, A., A.H. Bakhtiary, F. Elham and A. Rezasoltani. 2012. Effects of genu varum deformity on postural stability. *Int J Sports Med* 33 (6): 469-73.

Sorensen, K.L., M.A. Holland and E. Patla. 2002. The effects of human ankle muscle vibration on posture and balance during adaptive locomotion. *Exp Brain Res* 143 (1): 24-34.

Strecker, W., P. Keppler, F. Gebhard and L. Kinzl. 1997. Length and torsion of the lower limb. *J Bone Joint Surg Br* 79 (6): 1019-23.

Tinkle, B.T. *Issues and management of joint hypermobility.* 2008. Niles, IL: Left Paw Press.

Turner, M.S., and I.S. Smillie. 1981. The effect of tibial torsion on the pathology of the knee. *J Bone Joint Surg Br* 63-(B) (3): 396-98.

Vicenzino, B., M. Franettovich, T. McPoil, T. Russell, G. Skardoon and S. Bartold. 2005. Initial effects of antipronation tape on the medial longitudinal arch during walking and running. *Br J Sports Med* 39 (12): 939-43.

Whitman, R. 2010. The classic: A study of weak foot, with reference to its causes, its diagnosis, and its cure, with an analysis of a thousand cases of so-called flat-foot 1896. *Clin Orthop Relat Res.* 468 (4): 925-39.

Williams, D.S., I.S. McClay and J. Hamill. 2001. Arch structure and injury patterns in runners. *Clinical Biomech* (Bristol, Avon) 16 (4): 341-7.

Chapter 9

Ackermann, B., R. Adams, and A. Marshall. 2002. The effect of scapula taping on electromyographic activity and musical performance in professional violinists. *Australian Journal of Physiotherapy.* 28: 197-203.

Brunstromm, S. *Clinical kinesiology.* 2012. Eds P.A. Houglum and D.B. Bertoti. 6th ed. Philadelphia: Davis.

Cabrera, A.L., K.D. Plancher, S.C. Petterson and J.E. Kuhn. 2014. Treatment of medial and lateral scapular winging: Tendon transfers. *Oper Tech Sports Med* 22 (1): 97-107.

Cole, A.K., M.L. McGrath, S.E. Harrington, D.A. Padua, T.J. Rucinski and W.E Prentice. 2013. Scapular bracing and alteration in posture and muscle activity in overhead athletes with poor posture. *J Athl Train* 48 (1): 12-24.

Cools, A.N., V. Dewitte, F. Lanszweet, D. Notebaert, A. Roets, B. Soetens, B. Cagnie and E.E. Witvrouw. 2007. Rehabilitation of scapular muscle balance: Which exercises to prescribe? *American J of Sports Med* 35 (10): 1744-1751.

Culham, E., and M. Peat. 1993. Functional anatomy of the shoulder complex. *J Orthop Sports Phys Ther* 18 (1): 342-50.

DiVeta, J., M.L. Walker and B. Skibinski. 1990. Relationship between performance of selected scapular muscles and scapular abduction in standing subjects. *Phys Ther* 70 (8): 470-79.

Escamilla, R.F., K. Yamishiro, L. Paulos and J.R. Andrews. 2009. Shoulder muscle activity and function in common shoulder rehabilitation exercises. *Sports Med* 39 (8): 663-85.

Fitz, G.W. 1906. A clinical and anatomical study of resistant forward shoulders. *Boston Medical and Surgical Journal* 154: 423-31. DOI: 10.1056/NEJM190604191541601. Accessed September 2014.

Forthomme, B., J-M. Crielaard and J-L. Croisier. 2008. Scapular positioning in athlete's shoulder. *Sports Medicine* 38 (5): 369-86.

Greenfield, B., P.A. Catlin, P.W. Coats, E. Green, J.J. McDonald and C. North. 1995. Posture in patients with shoulder overuse injuries and healthy individuals. *J Orthop Sports Phys Ther* 21 (5): 287-95.

Hoppenfeld, S. 1976. *Physical examination of the spine and extremities.* New York: Appleton-Century Crafts.

Kendall, F.P., E.K. McCreary and P.G. Provance. 1993. *Muscles: Testing and function.* 4th ed. Baltimore: Lippincott Williams and Wilkins.

Kibler, W.B., P.M. Ludewig, P.W. McClure, L.A. Michener, K. Bak and A.D. Sciacia. 2013. Clinical implications of scapula dyskinesis in shoulder injury: The 2013 consensus statement from the scapular summit. *British Journal of Sports Medicine* 47 (2013): 877-85. DOI: 10.1136/bjsports-2013-092425. Accessed September 2014.

Klebe, T.M., K.V. Døssing, T. Blenstrup, J. Nielsen-Ferreira, L. Rejsenhus, G. Aalkjaer and M. Breddam. 2003. Scapulae alatae—angels' wings. A study of 64 patients treated with braces and physical therapy at the Viberg's hospital. *Ugeskr Laeger* 165 (17): 1779-82.

Levangie, P.K., and C.C. Norkin. 2001. *Joint structure and function: A comprehensive analysis*. Philadelphia: Davis.

Lewis, J.S., C. Wright and A. Green. 2005. Subacromial impingement syndrome: The effect of changing posture on shoulder range of movement. *J Orthop Sports Phys Ther* 35 (2): 72-87.

Magee, D.J. 2002. *Orthopedic physical assessment.* 4th ed. Philadelphia: Saunders.

Martin, R.M., and D.E. Fish. 2008. Scapular winging: Anatomical review, diagnosis and treatments. *Curr Rev Musculoskelet Med* 1 (1): 1–11.

Meininger, A.K., B.F. Figuerres and B.A. Goldberg. 2011. Scapular winging: An update. *J M Acad Orthop Surg* 19 (8): 453-62.

Oyama, S., J.B. Myers, C.A. Wessinger, R.D. Ricci and S.M Lephart. 2008. Asymmetric resting scapular posture in healthy overhead athletes. *J of Athletic Training* 43 (6): 565-70.

Smith, J., T.D. Dietrich, B.R. Kotajarvi and K.R. Kaufman. 2006. The effect of scapular protraction on isometric shoulder rotator strength in normal subjects. *J Shoulder Elbow Surg* 15 (3): 339-43.

Sobush, D.C., G.G. Simoneau, K.E. Dietz, J.A. Levene, R.E. Grossman and W.B. Smith. 1996. The Lennie test for measuring scapula position in healthy young adult females: A reliability and validity study. *J Orthop Sports Phys Ther* 23 (1): 39-50.

Tibaek, S. and J. Gadsboell. 2014. Scapula alata: Description of a physical therapy program and its effectiveness measured by a shoulder-specific quality-of-life measurement. *J Shoulder Elbow Surg* 1-9.. www.jshoulderelbow.org/article/S1058-2746(14)00388-7/abstract. Accessed December 2014.

Chapter 10

Alter, M.J. 2004. *The science of flexibility*. Champaign, IL: Human Kinetics.

American Academy of Orthopaedic Surgeons (W.B. Greene and J.D. Heckman, Eds). 1994. *Clinical measurement of joint motion*. Rosemont (IL).

Jacobs, C.A., and A.D. Sciascia. 2011. Factors that influence the efficacy of stretching programmes for patients with hypomobility. *Sports Health* 3 (6): 520-23.

Kaux, J.F., B. Forthomme, M. Foldart-Dessalle, F. Delvaux, F.G. Debray, J.M. Crielaard and J.L. Crosier. 2013. Eccentric training for elbow hypermobility. *Journal of Novel Physiotherapies* 3 (6): 180. DOI: 10.4172/2165-7025.1000180. Accessed December 2014,

Kirk, J.A., B.M. Ansell and E.G. Bywaters. 1967. The hypermobility syndrome: Musculoskeletal complaints associated with generalized hypermobility. *Ann Rheu. Dis* 26 (5): 419-25.

Levangie, P.K., and C.C. Norkin. 2001. *Joint structure and function: A comprehensive analysis*. Philadelphia: Davis.

MacKay-Lyons, M. 1989. Low-load prolonged stretch in treatment of elbow flexion contractures secondary to head trauma: A case report. *Phys Ther* 69 (4): 292-96.

Magee, D.J. 2002. *Orthopedic physical assessment.* 4th ed. Philadelphia: Saunders.

Morrey, B.F., L.J. Askew and E.Y. Chao. 1981. A biomechanical study of normal functional elbow motion. *J Bone Joint Surg Am* 36 (6): 872-7.

Müller, A.M., P. Sadoghi, R. Lucas, L. Audige, R. Delany, M. Klein, V. Valderrabano and P. Vavken. 2013. Effectiveness of bracing in the treatment of nonoseesoes restriction of elbow mobility: A systematic review and meta-analysis of 13 studies. *J Shoulder Elbow Surg* 22 (8): 1146-52.

Nandi, S., S. Maschke, P.J. Evans and J.N. Lawton. 2009. The stiff elbow. *Hand (N Y)* 4 (4): 368-79.

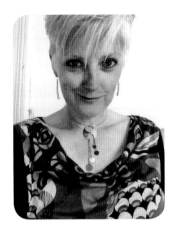

Jane Johnson, MSc, is a chartered physiotherapist and sport massage therapist specializing in occupational health. In this role she spends much time assessing the posture of clients and examining whether work, sport, or recreational postures may be contributing to their symptoms. She devises postural correction plans that include both hands-on and hands-off techniques.

Johnson has taught continuing professional development (CPD) workshops for many organizations both in the UK and abroad. This experience has brought her into contact with thousands of therapists of all disciplines and informed her own practice. She is passionate about supporting and inspiring newly qualified or less confident therapists so they feel more self-assured in their work.

Johnson is a member of the Chartered Society of Physiotherapy and is registered with the Health Professions Council. A member of the Medico Legal Association of Chartered Physiotherapists, she provides expert witness reports on cases involving soft tissue therapies.

In her spare time, Johnson enjoys taking her dog for long walks, sketching and visiting museums. She resides in northeast England.

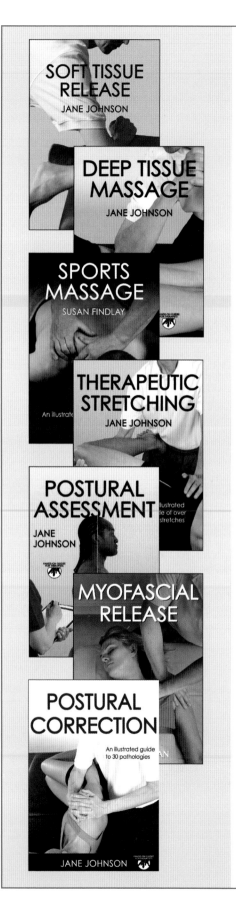

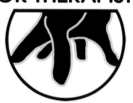
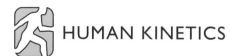